# Personal Approach to Patient Care

# A Personal Approach to Patient Care

P. J. Hunt
B. Sendell

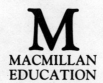

MACMILLAN
EDUCATION

First published 1987

Published by
MACMILLAN EDUCATION LTD
Houndmills, Basingstoke, Hampshire RG21 2XS
and London
Companies and representatives
throughout the world

Typeset and designed by
Oxprint Ltd., Oxford
Printed in Great Britain by Scotprint Ltd., Musselburgh

British Library Cataloguing in Publication Data
Hunt, Patricia
A personal approach to patient care.
1. Nursing
I. Title    II. Sendell, Bernice
610.73        RT41
ISBN 0–333–40862–4 Pbk

To the patients of the reader

# Contents

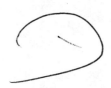

Foreword                                    vi
Preface                                     vii
Acknowledgements                            viii

**Section 1    Needs**                      **1**

1       Identification of Needs             3
2       Differences in Individuals          10


**Section 2    The Patient**                **41**

3       Breathing                           42
4       Eating and Drinking                 76
5       Eliminating                         110
6       Sleeping and Resting                156
7       Multiple Living Activities          184


**Section 3    The Nurse**                  **225**

8       The Roles of the Nurse              226

*Postscript: Rule of Conduct*               235

# Foreword

The diversity of nursing and the increasing number of specialist groups it contains often makes for confusion in observers, its own practitioners and in aspiring members of the profession. This book sets out a concept of basic care which underpins the wide variety of nursing activities. It provides a critical framework which enables the nurse to adapt this care to meet specific individual needs. In so doing, it provides not only a setting within which learner and practitioner alike can develop and extend their professional practice, but it also demonstrates the underlying principles of care which are the keystone to the profession of nursing.

M. W. Watson, BSc, SRN, SCM
*Director of Nurse Education*
*Bristol and Weston School of Nursing*

# Preface

We have great pleasure in introducing this nursing text which we hope will be useful and give opportunity for discussion to all nurses and nursing students. We have divided the book into three major sections. The first section gives guidance as to how people differ in response to growth, development, ageing, temperament, social and cultural influences and individual mental and physical capacity. We identify four major categories of needs and give examples of how these may be satisfied.

In the second section we have used Virginia Henderson's components of basic nursing and have looked at functions that require assistance. Each of the five chapters gives references for revision of normal physiology, then consideration is given to the social and psychological factors affecting the chosen living activity. This is followed by a patient history with guidance for assessing the patient's needs, choosing priorities in nursing care and setting short- and long-term goals. At the end of each chapter is a selection of further medical and surgical conditions which may affect living activities, with further reading of selected aspects of pharmacology, physiotherapy and nursing procedures.

The third section considers the multiple roles of the nurse and asks some pertinent questions which could be used for self-evaluation and further activity.

Throughout the complete text the emphasis is on encouraging the reader to participate and in so doing develop a systematic way of assessing, planning and evaluating care.

1987

P. J. H.
B. S.

## A NOTE TO THE READER

We would like to emphasise that each patient regardless of age, temperament or social/cultural background is first and foremost an individual. There can be no substitute for reaching an understanding of the individual patient. This book can only be a very general guide which offers some clues to help you towards that understanding.

A comment from a patient:
*'What kind of people do they think we are?'*

# Acknowledgements

The authors would like to extend their thanks to the following people: Wendy Watson, Director of Nurse Education, Bristol and Weston School of Nursing, for her understanding support; Alice Henley for her versatility and willingness in typing our manuscript; Shirley Stephen and Anne Lawrence, Librarians, and their supporting staff at the Bristol and Weston School of Nursing for their assistance; Elizabeth Horne, previously Nursing Editor at Macmillan Press, for continuing encouragement; Anne Betts for reading our efforts and giving constructive criticism; and all the students and staff who have provided feedback prior to publication.

# Section 1   Needs

## Introduction

Within this text you will find an opportunity to consider how people differ and alter in response to growth, development, ageing, temperament, social and cultural influences and individual physical and mental capacity. Superimposed on this normal way of life are the changes which can occur in ill-health and when there is reduced ability to maintain physiological, security, achievement and self-fulfilment needs.

You will be asked to carry out activities throughout the text to enable you to apply the principles discussed.

Chapter 1 starts by considering the needs of an individual and then explores the ever-present factors that affect these needs, such as age and temperament. This forms a basis for the consideration of a nursing model of care. We then discuss in detail how these models vary and how they can be used to assist patients/clients in carrying out living activites that will enable them to maintain physiological, security, achievement and self-fulfilment needs.

# Chapter 1

# Identification of Needs

If the concept of all people having needs, desires and interests which are fundamental to the physiological and psychological well-being of the individual is recognised then we can look at needs as described by psychologists and see how they can be used as a basis for nursing.

We are going to look at two different ways in which needs have been described (Maslow, 1968 and Adcock, 1969), and from these to choose a simple framework to enable you to discover how your present needs are satisfied and when they may be in jeopardy. By undertaking this activity you should be able to recognise how your physiological and psychological needs are satisfied and then be more able to identify how and when people's needs are fulfilled or put in danger.

Maslow identified a hierarchy of needs in which he stated that the lower physiological needs such as hunger and thirst had to be satisfied before the individual would consider seeking a secure and safe environment. Again the safety needs had to be satisfied before the needs for belonging and friends, until eventually the individual finds the climax which is self-actualisation, that is, he or she reaches self-fulfilment and individual potential. See *Figure 1.1*.

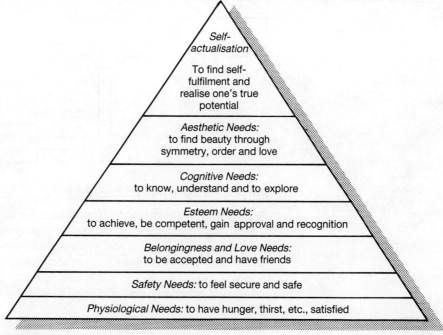

**Figure 1.1** *Maslow's hierarchy of needs*

Adcock discusses drives and needs of individuals, firstly, by identifying the biological and physiological drives and needs and, secondly, by looking at psychological and emergency drives and needs.

He identifies the need to satisfy hunger and the need for air as prime physiological needs, with other physiological requirements, to excrete, relieve fatigue and obtain sleep and rest, as essential for the individual. He then considers other needs with related drives, the sex and parental drives. The psychological needs and drives are identified as being the need for security and affection; the need to satisfy curiosity and to know and understand; and the need for aesthetic and sensory satisfaction.

In order for the individual to adjust to changes in the environment other energy drives such as anger, fear and excitement are mobilised to ensure that the individual copes with the situation.

Adcock states that needs are closely interrelated with particular need for security and achievement but in no way does he suggest the hierarchical nature of Maslow's description. See *Figure 1.2*.

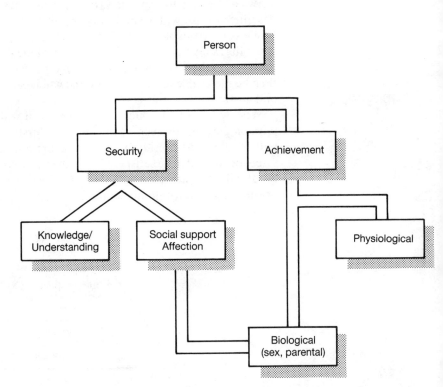

**Figure 1.2** *The interrelation of needs*

We accept that there is a theoretical basis for the identification of fundamental needs and requirements which are common to all individuals and are essential for self-fulfilment and attainment of potential.

There are possibly as many ways of identifying and classifying needs as there are psychologists and you may wish now to pause and explore suitable psychology textbooks such as those by E. R. Hilgard (1971) and J. A. C. Brown (1964).

We have therefore chosen to divide the multiplicity of needs which have been identified into four categories and these are outlined in *Table 1.1*.

*Table 1.1    Four categories of needs*

| 1. Physiological | The need for |
|---|---|
| | ● air |
| | ● food and water |
| | ● shelter |
| | ● exercise |
| | ● sleep and rest |
| | ● elimination |
| 2. Security needs | The need for |
| | ● safety |
| | ● affection |
| | ● belonging |
| 3. Achievement needs | The need for |
| | ● approval |
| | ● respect |
| | ● dignity |
| 4. Self-fulfilment needs | The need for |
| | ● knowledge |
| | ● aesthetic and sensory satisfaction |
| | ● realisation of potential |

Physiological needs are largely satisfied by daily living activities such as breathing, eating and drinking, living in a comfortable home, having time and place for suitable rest, sleep and elimination.

The security needs are dependent for their satisfaction on living in a safe environment with the affection of others, and belonging and communicating with a group, family unit and/or community.

In order to have a sense of achievement an individual requires the approval and respect of others and to be treated with dignity and understanding of his/her attainments.

To become a complete individual the self-fulfilment need has to be satisfied by the knowledge gained through curiosity and explanation by aesthetic and sensory enjoyment and by realisation of individual potential.

For example, within our society most people satisfy their physiological needs by living in a clean air environment, not smoking, living at or near sea level, buying or growing and cooking their own food, eating and drinking without assistance, eliminating in privacy, living in a warm, dry, secure home and regulating their activities, and providing time for adequate exercise, rest and sleep. To satisfy this need for security most people take steps to ensure a safe environment within their place of residence, work, school, or leisure activity. They gain a sense of belonging and affection from their immediate family and friends, and by belonging to groups, societies and communities.

To meet achievement needs most people have approval for their actions from friends and relations, gain respect from colleagues and team members and preserve their dignity by the support of others. Self-fulfilment needs can be met by the person seeking knowledge through curiosity and discovery, by gaining aesthetic and sensory satisfaction from enjoyment through seeing, hearing, touching, smelling and tasting, and by having the mental and physical capacity to realise individual potential in the context of work or leisure or living activities.

You may now find it useful to consider how your needs are being satisfied at present. *Table 1.2* is a questionnaire designed to help you.

Table 1.2    Questionnaire: How are your needs satisfied?

| 1. **PHYSIOLOGICAL NEEDS** How do you satisfy your need for the following: | |
| --- | --- |
| ● air | |
| ● food | |
| ● drink | |
| ● elimination | |
| ● shelter | |
| ● exercise | |

| | |
|---|---|
| ● rest | |
| ● sleep? | |
| 2. **SECURITY NEEDS**<br>How do you satisfy your<br>need for: | |
| ● safety at home | |
| ● safety at school/work | |
| ● safety at leisure | |
| ● affection | |
| ● sense of belonging? | |
| 3. **ACHIEVEMENT NEEDS**<br>From whom do you seek | |
| ● approval | |

*Table 1.2 Continued*

| | |
|---|---|
| ● respect? | |
| How do you maintain your dignity?<br><br>What would you find a threat to your dignity? | |
| **4. SELF-FULFILMENT NEEDS**<br>How do you gain new knowledge? | |
| What activities do you most enjoy? Those involving:<br>● what you see<br>● what you hear<br>● what you touch<br>● what you taste/smell | |
| How do you know when you have reached the limits of your capabilities<br>● at work<br>● at school<br>● at leisure? | |
| How many of the foregoing activities have you given up and which are you still pursuing? | |

You may like to try this questionnaire on one of your friends/neighbours/relatives and compare how the same needs may be satisfied in a different manner.

Having now had practice at using the four main groups of needs as a framework for looking at the individual we will start to study the factors or characteristics that affect the ways in which needs may be satisfied. These factors are:

● your age
● your temperament
● your social/cultural environment
● your mental and physical capacity.

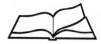

## REFERENCES

Adcock, C. J. (1969). *Fundamentals of Psychology*. Pelican Books, Harmondsworth, Middx.

Brown, J. A. C. (1964). *Freud and the Post-Freudians*. Penguin Books, Harmondsworth, Middx.

Hilgard, E. R. *et al.* (1971). *Introduction to Psychology*. Harcourt Brace Jovanovich, New York.

Maslow, A. H. (1968). *Towards a Psychology of Being*. Van Nostrand Reinhold, New York.

# *Chapter 2*
# **Differences in Individuals**

In this chapter we shall consider how age, temperament, social/cultural environment and mental and physical capacity can affect the ways in which needs are satisfied. This will further your understanding of the differences in individuals. To do this you will find a series of profiles from which you will be able to compare individuals' abilities to satisfy their own needs and be able to identify when assistance is required from others. You should start at the top right-hand section of the profile and continue in a clockwise direction as shown in *Figure 2.1*.

You need to remember that these profiles are only guidelines and that everyone is an individual and may respond differently to the 'normal' profile.

**Figure 2.1**  *Patient profile*

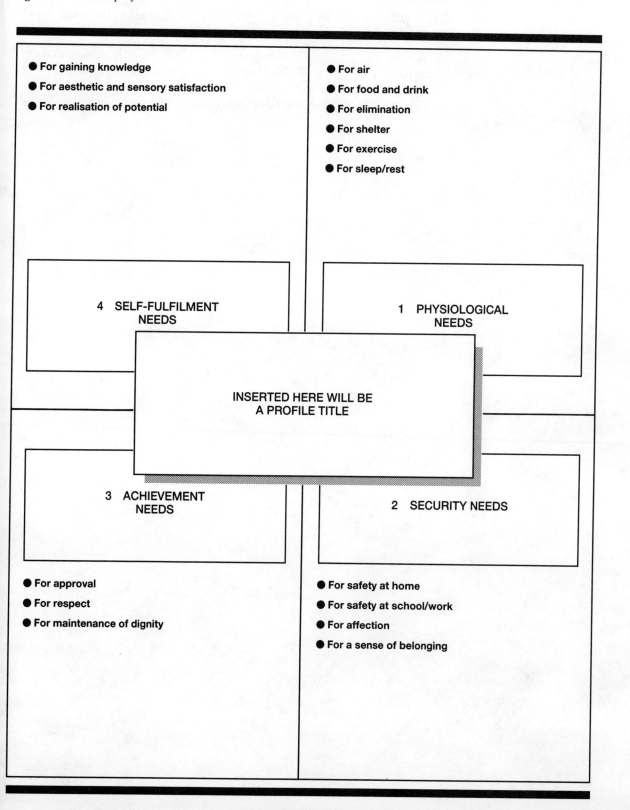

- For gaining knowledge
- For aesthetic and sensory satisfaction
- For realisation of potential

- For air
- For food and drink
- For elimination
- For shelter
- For exercise
- For sleep/rest

4   SELF-FULFILMENT
NEEDS

1   PHYSIOLOGICAL
NEEDS

INSERTED HERE WILL BE
A PROFILE TITLE

3   ACHIEVEMENT
NEEDS

2   SECURITY NEEDS

- For approval
- For respect
- For maintenance of dignity

- For safety at home
- For safety at school/work
- For affection
- For a sense of belonging

## EFFECT OF AGE

Here are some chosen profiles to show how *age* can affect the ways in which needs are satisfied. As examples we have chosen:

1. A baby
2. A toddler
3. Early school age
4. Eleven-year-old

5. Adolescent
6. Mid-twenties
7. Mid-life 35–45 years
8. Pre-retirement

9. Early post-retirement
10. Eighty-year-old

**Figure 2.2**  *A baby profile*

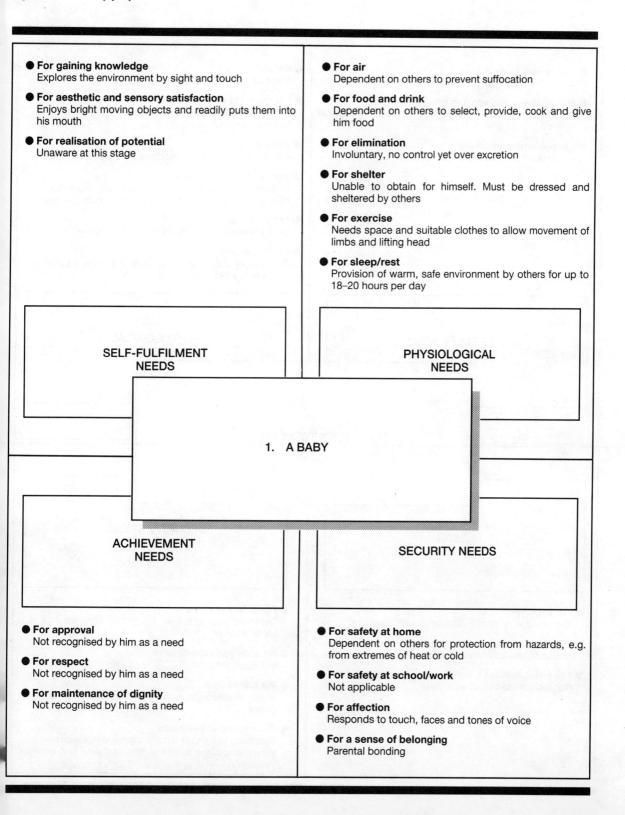

**Figure 2.3**  *A toddler profile*

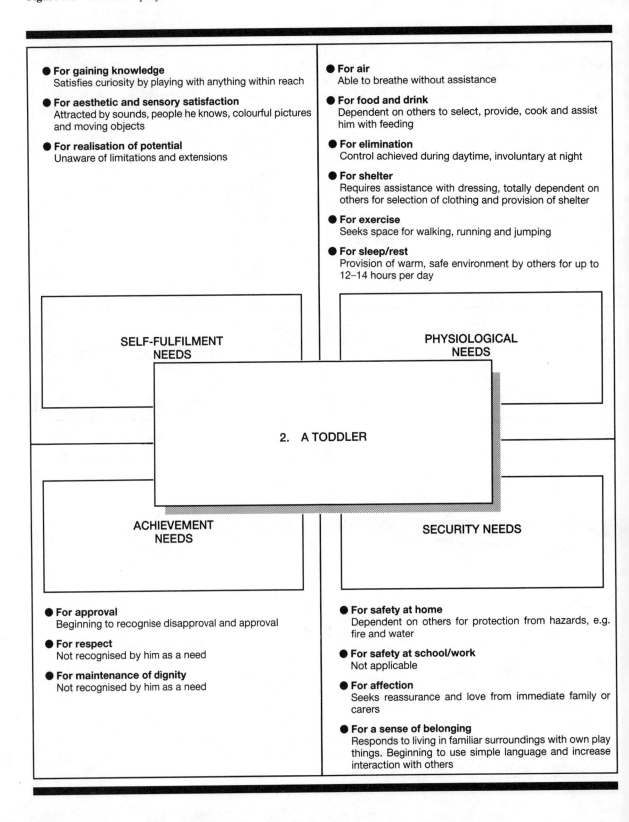

● **For gaining knowledge**
Satisfies curiosity by playing with anything within reach

● **For aesthetic and sensory satisfaction**
Attracted by sounds, people he knows, colourful pictures and moving objects

● **For realisation of potential**
Unaware of limitations and extensions

● **For air**
Able to breathe without assistance

● **For food and drink**
Dependent on others to select, provide, cook and assist him with feeding

● **For elimination**
Control achieved during daytime, involuntary at night

● **For shelter**
Requires assistance with dressing, totally dependent on others for selection of clothing and provision of shelter

● **For exercise**
Seeks space for walking, running and jumping

● **For sleep/rest**
Provision of warm, safe environment by others for up to 12–14 hours per day

**SELF-FULFILMENT NEEDS**

**PHYSIOLOGICAL NEEDS**

**2.    A TODDLER**

**ACHIEVEMENT NEEDS**

**SECURITY NEEDS**

● **For approval**
Beginning to recognise disapproval and approval

● **For respect**
Not recognised by him as a need

● **For maintenance of dignity**
Not recognised by him as a need

● **For safety at home**
Dependent on others for protection from hazards, e.g. fire and water

● **For safety at school/work**
Not applicable

● **For affection**
Seeks reassurance and love from immediate family or carers

● **For a sense of belonging**
Responds to living in familiar surroundings with own play things. Beginning to use simple language and increase interaction with others

**Figure 2.4**  *Early school age profile*

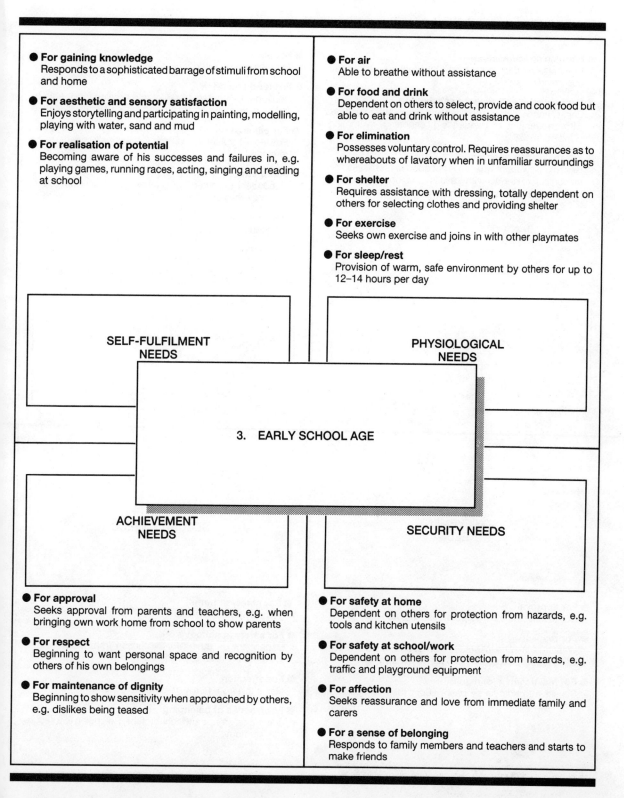

● **For gaining knowledge**
Responds to a sophisticated barrage of stimuli from school and home

● **For aesthetic and sensory satisfaction**
Enjoys storytelling and participating in painting, modelling, playing with water, sand and mud

● **For realisation of potential**
Becoming aware of his successes and failures in, e.g. playing games, running races, acting, singing and reading at school

● **For air**
Able to breathe without assistance

● **For food and drink**
Dependent on others to select, provide and cook food but able to eat and drink without assistance

● **For elimination**
Possesses voluntary control. Requires reassurances as to whereabouts of lavatory when in unfamiliar surroundings

● **For shelter**
Requires assistance with dressing, totally dependent on others for selecting clothes and providing shelter

● **For exercise**
Seeks own exercise and joins in with other playmates

● **For sleep/rest**
Provision of warm, safe environment by others for up to 12–14 hours per day

SELF-FULFILMENT
NEEDS

PHYSIOLOGICAL
NEEDS

3.   EARLY SCHOOL AGE

ACHIEVEMENT
NEEDS

SECURITY NEEDS

● **For approval**
Seeks approval from parents and teachers, e.g. when bringing own work home from school to show parents

● **For respect**
Beginning to want personal space and recognition by others of his own belongings

● **For maintenance of dignity**
Beginning to show sensitivity when approached by others, e.g. dislikes being teased

● **For safety at home**
Dependent on others for protection from hazards, e.g. tools and kitchen utensils

● **For safety at school/work**
Dependent on others for protection from hazards, e.g. traffic and playground equipment

● **For affection**
Seeks reassurance and love from immediate family and carers

● **For a sense of belonging**
Responds to family members and teachers and starts to make friends

**Figure 2.5**    *Eleven-year-old profile*

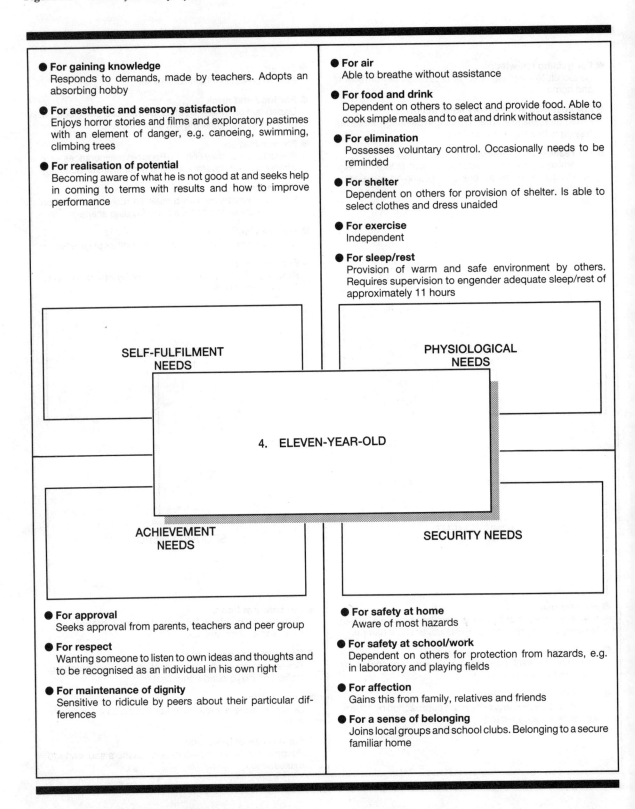

● **For gaining knowledge**
Responds to demands, made by teachers. Adopts an absorbing hobby

● **For aesthetic and sensory satisfaction**
Enjoys horror stories and films and exploratory pastimes with an element of danger, e.g. canoeing, swimming, climbing trees

● **For realisation of potential**
Becoming aware of what he is not good at and seeks help in coming to terms with results and how to improve performance

● **For air**
Able to breathe without assistance

● **For food and drink**
Dependent on others to select and provide food. Able to cook simple meals and to eat and drink without assistance

● **For elimination**
Possesses voluntary control. Occasionally needs to be reminded

● **For shelter**
Dependent on others for provision of shelter. Is able to select clothes and dress unaided

● **For exercise**
Independent

● **For sleep/rest**
Provision of warm and safe environment by others. Requires supervision to engender adequate sleep/rest of approximately 11 hours

SELF-FULFILMENT
NEEDS

PHYSIOLOGICAL
NEEDS

4.    ELEVEN-YEAR-OLD

ACHIEVEMENT
NEEDS

SECURITY NEEDS

● **For approval**
Seeks approval from parents, teachers and peer group

● **For respect**
Wanting someone to listen to own ideas and thoughts and to be recognised as an individual in his own right

● **For maintenance of dignity**
Sensitive to ridicule by peers about their particular differences

● **For safety at home**
Aware of most hazards

● **For safety at school/work**
Dependent on others for protection from hazards, e.g. in laboratory and playing fields

● **For affection**
Gains this from family, relatives and friends

● **For a sense of belonging**
Joins local groups and school clubs. Belonging to a secure familiar home

**Figure 2.6**  *Adolescent profile*

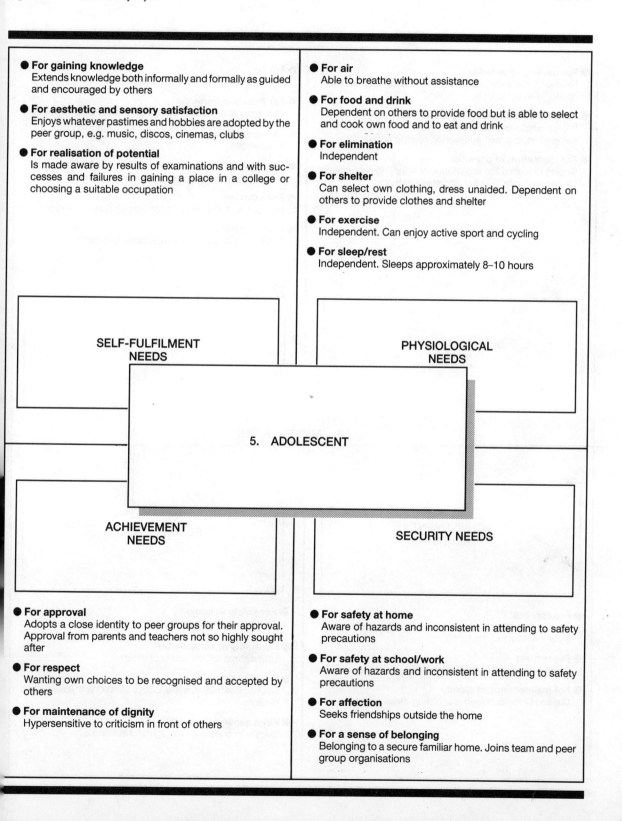

**For gaining knowledge**
Extends knowledge both informally and formally as guided and encouraged by others

**For aesthetic and sensory satisfaction**
Enjoys whatever pastimes and hobbies are adopted by the peer group, e.g. music, discos, cinemas, clubs

**For realisation of potential**
Is made aware by results of examinations and with successes and failures in gaining a place in a college or choosing a suitable occupation

**For air**
Able to breathe without assistance

**For food and drink**
Dependent on others to provide food but is able to select and cook own food and to eat and drink

**For elimination**
Independent

**For shelter**
Can select own clothing, dress unaided. Dependent on others to provide clothes and shelter

**For exercise**
Independent. Can enjoy active sport and cycling

**For sleep/rest**
Independent. Sleeps approximately 8–10 hours

**SELF-FULFILMENT NEEDS**

**PHYSIOLOGICAL NEEDS**

**5.   ADOLESCENT**

**ACHIEVEMENT NEEDS**

**SECURITY NEEDS**

**For approval**
Adopts a close identity to peer groups for their approval. Approval from parents and teachers not so highly sought after

**For respect**
Wanting own choices to be recognised and accepted by others

**For maintenance of dignity**
Hypersensitive to criticism in front of others

**For safety at home**
Aware of hazards and inconsistent in attending to safety precautions

**For safety at school/work**
Aware of hazards and inconsistent in attending to safety precautions

**For affection**
Seeks friendships outside the home

**For a sense of belonging**
Belonging to a secure familiar home. Joins team and peer group organisations

**Figure 2.7**   *Mid-twenties profile*

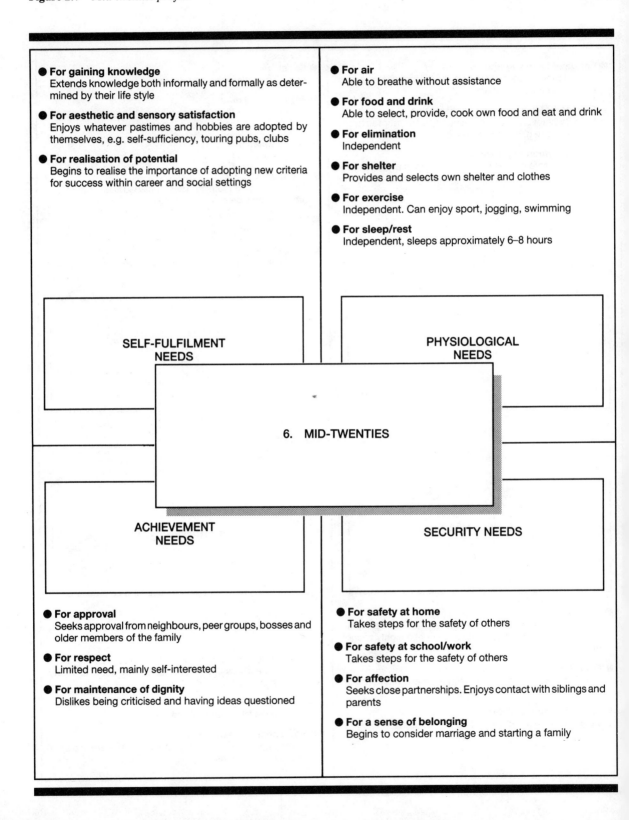

● **For gaining knowledge**
Extends knowledge both informally and formally as determined by their life style

● **For aesthetic and sensory satisfaction**
Enjoys whatever pastimes and hobbies are adopted by
themselves, e.g. self-sufficiency, touring pubs, clubs

● **For realisation of potential**
Begins to realise the importance of adopting new criteria
for success within career and social settings

● **For air**
Able to breathe without assistance

● **For food and drink**
Able to select, provide, cook own food and eat and drink

● **For elimination**
Independent

● **For shelter**
Provides and selects own shelter and clothes

● **For exercise**
Independent. Can enjoy sport, jogging, swimming

● **For sleep/rest**
Independent, sleeps approximately 6–8 hours

**SELF-FULFILMENT
NEEDS**

**PHYSIOLOGICAL
NEEDS**

**6.   MID-TWENTIES**

**ACHIEVEMENT
NEEDS**

**SECURITY NEEDS**

● **For approval**
Seeks approval from neighbours, peer groups, bosses and
older members of the family

● **For respect**
Limited need, mainly self-interested

● **For maintenance of dignity**
Dislikes being criticised and having ideas questioned

● **For safety at home**
Takes steps for the safety of others

● **For safety at school/work**
Takes steps for the safety of others

● **For affection**
Seeks close partnerships. Enjoys contact with siblings and
parents

● **For a sense of belonging**
Begins to consider marriage and starting a family

**Figure 2.8**   *Mid-life profile*

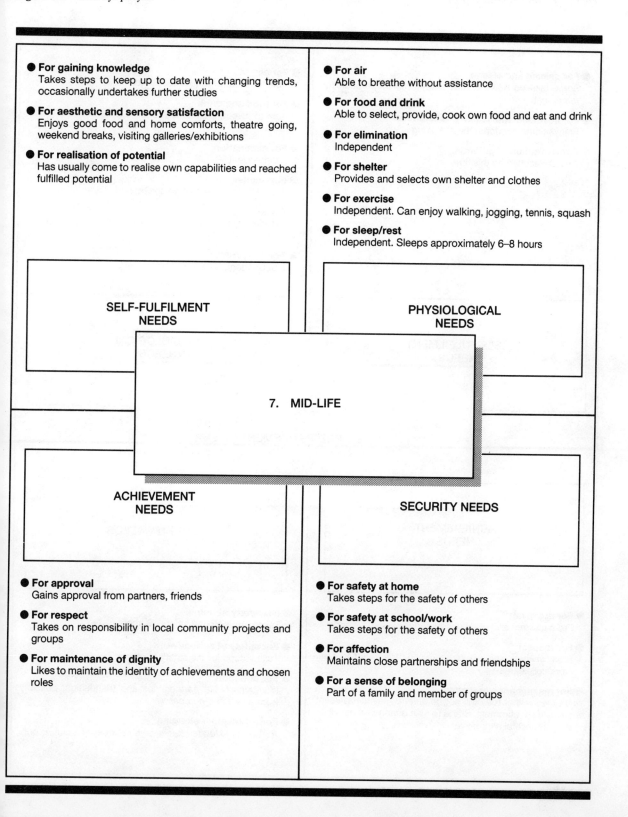

● **For gaining knowledge**
Takes steps to keep up to date with changing trends, occasionally undertakes further studies

● **For aesthetic and sensory satisfaction**
Enjoys good food and home comforts, theatre going, weekend breaks, visiting galleries/exhibitions

● **For realisation of potential**
Has usually come to realise own capabilities and reached fulfilled potential

● **For air**
Able to breathe without assistance

● **For food and drink**
Able to select, provide, cook own food and eat and drink

● **For elimination**
Independent

● **For shelter**
Provides and selects own shelter and clothes

● **For exercise**
Independent. Can enjoy walking, jogging, tennis, squash

● **For sleep/rest**
Independent. Sleeps approximately 6–8 hours

SELF-FULFILMENT
NEEDS

PHYSIOLOGICAL
NEEDS

7.   MID-LIFE

ACHIEVEMENT
NEEDS

SECURITY NEEDS

● **For approval**
Gains approval from partners, friends

● **For respect**
Takes on responsibility in local community projects and groups

● **For maintenance of dignity**
Likes to maintain the identity of achievements and chosen roles

● **For safety at home**
Takes steps for the safety of others

● **For safety at school/work**
Takes steps for the safety of others

● **For affection**
Maintains close partnerships and friendships

● **For a sense of belonging**
Part of a family and member of groups

**Figure 2.9**  *Pre-retirement profile*

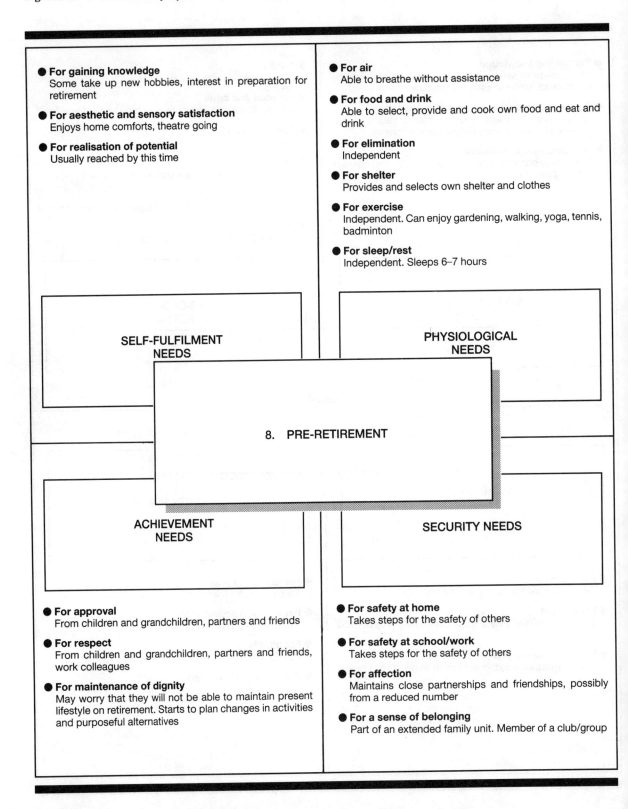

● **For gaining knowledge**
Some take up new hobbies, interest in preparation for retirement

● **For aesthetic and sensory satisfaction**
Enjoys home comforts, theatre going

● **For realisation of potential**
Usually reached by this time

● **For air**
Able to breathe without assistance

● **For food and drink**
Able to select, provide and cook own food and eat and drink

● **For elimination**
Independent

● **For shelter**
Provides and selects own shelter and clothes

● **For exercise**
Independent. Can enjoy gardening, walking, yoga, tennis, badminton

● **For sleep/rest**
Independent. Sleeps 6–7 hours

SELF-FULFILMENT
NEEDS

PHYSIOLOGICAL
NEEDS

8.   PRE-RETIREMENT

ACHIEVEMENT
NEEDS

SECURITY NEEDS

● **For approval**
From children and grandchildren, partners and friends

● **For respect**
From children and grandchildren, partners and friends, work colleagues

● **For maintenance of dignity**
May worry that they will not be able to maintain present lifestyle on retirement. Starts to plan changes in activities and purposeful alternatives

● **For safety at home**
Takes steps for the safety of others

● **For safety at school/work**
Takes steps for the safety of others

● **For affection**
Maintains close partnerships and friendships, possibly from a reduced number

● **For a sense of belonging**
Part of an extended family unit. Member of a club/group

**Figure 2.10**  *Early post-retirement profile*

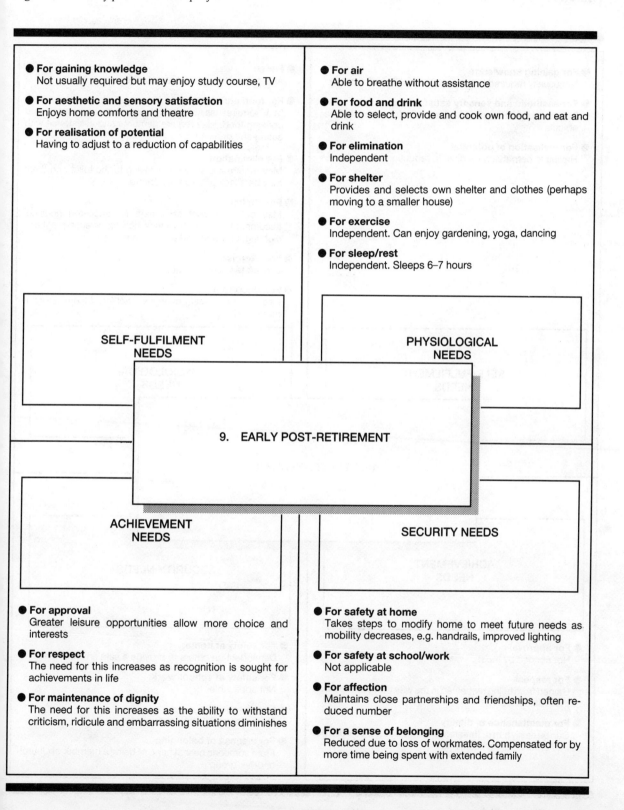

● **For gaining knowledge**
Not usually required but may enjoy study course, TV

● **For aesthetic and sensory satisfaction**
Enjoys home comforts and theatre

● **For realisation of potential**
Having to adjust to a reduction of capabilities

● **For air**
Able to breathe without assistance

● **For food and drink**
Able to select, provide and cook own food, and eat and drink

● **For elimination**
Independent

● **For shelter**
Provides and selects own shelter and clothes (perhaps moving to a smaller house)

● **For exercise**
Independent. Can enjoy gardening, yoga, dancing

● **For sleep/rest**
Independent. Sleeps 6–7 hours

**SELF-FULFILMENT NEEDS**

**PHYSIOLOGICAL NEEDS**

**9.  EARLY POST-RETIREMENT**

**ACHIEVEMENT NEEDS**

**SECURITY NEEDS**

● **For approval**
Greater leisure opportunities allow more choice and interests

● **For respect**
The need for this increases as recognition is sought for achievements in life

● **For maintenance of dignity**
The need for this increases as the ability to withstand criticism, ridicule and embarrassing situations diminishes

● **For safety at home**
Takes steps to modify home to meet future needs as mobility decreases, e.g. handrails, improved lighting

● **For safety at school/work**
Not applicable

● **For affection**
Maintains close partnerships and friendships, often reduced number

● **For a sense of belonging**
Reduced due to loss of workmates. Compensated for by more time being spent with extended family

**Figure 2.11**  *Eighty-year-old profile*

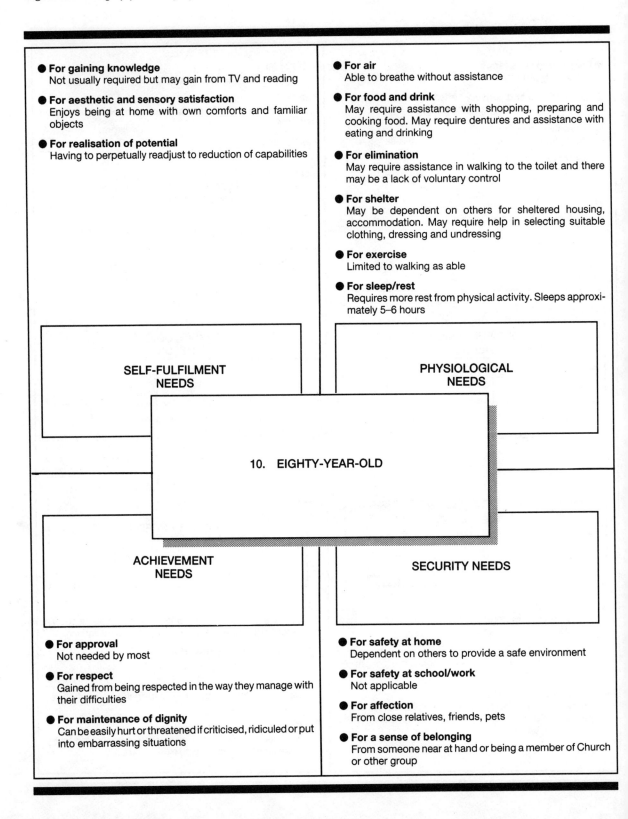

● **For gaining knowledge**
Not usually required but may gain from TV and reading

● **For aesthetic and sensory satisfaction**
Enjoys being at home with own comforts and familiar objects

● **For realisation of potential**
Having to perpetually readjust to reduction of capabilities

● **For air**
Able to breathe without assistance

● **For food and drink**
May require assistance with shopping, preparing and cooking food. May require dentures and assistance with eating and drinking

● **For elimination**
May require assistance in walking to the toilet and there may be a lack of voluntary control

● **For shelter**
May be dependent on others for sheltered housing, accommodation. May require help in selecting suitable clothing, dressing and undressing

● **For exercise**
Limited to walking as able

● **For sleep/rest**
Requires more rest from physical activity. Sleeps approximately 5–6 hours

**SELF-FULFILMENT NEEDS**

**PHYSIOLOGICAL NEEDS**

**10.   EIGHTY-YEAR-OLD**

**ACHIEVEMENT NEEDS**

**SECURITY NEEDS**

● **For approval**
Not needed by most

● **For respect**
Gained from being respected in the way they manage with their difficulties

● **For maintenance of dignity**
Can be easily hurt or threatened if criticised, ridiculed or put into embarrassing situations

● **For safety at home**
Dependent on others to provide a safe environment

● **For safety at school/work**
Not applicable

● **For affection**
From close relatives, friends, pets

● **For a sense of belonging**
From someone near at hand or being a member of Church or other group

**EFFECTS OF TEMPERAMENT**

Here are some chosen profiles to show how temperament can affect the ways in which needs are satisfied.

> 'The word temperament has long been used to describe differences in emotionality; we say of one person that he is even tempered, of another that he is quick to "fly off the handle". Such terms describe emotionality that is the readiness to experience and express emotional responses of various kinds. Persisting individual differences of this kind are considered to be aspects of personality.' (Hilgard *et al.*, 1953)

As examples we have chosen:

11. A person with a consistent increase in emotional response causing hyperactivity, aggression, irritability, fear, anxiety and/or euphoria (*Figure 2.12*).
12. A person with a consistent decrease in emotional response causing underactivity, depression, lack of spontaneity (*Figure 2.13*).

**Figure 2.12**    *Hyperactive person profile*

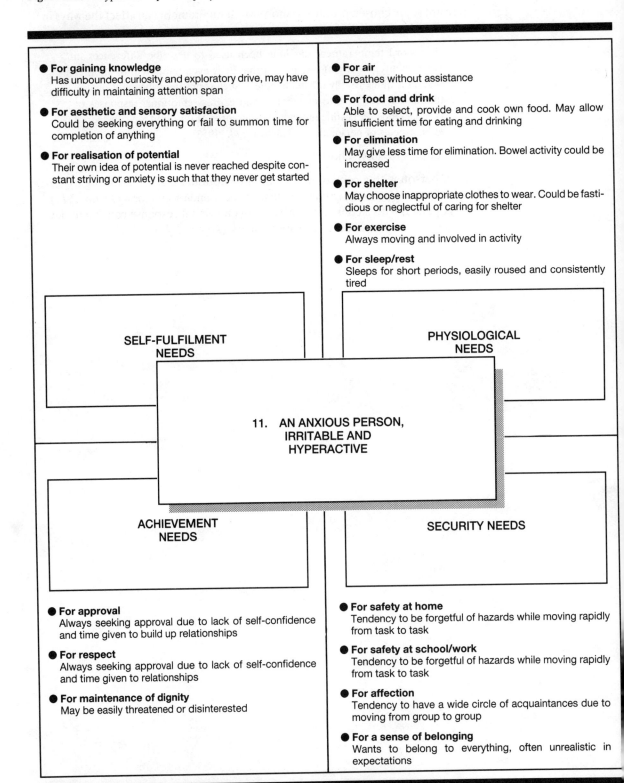

● **For gaining knowledge**
Has unbounded curiosity and exploratory drive, may have difficulty in maintaining attention span

● **For aesthetic and sensory satisfaction**
Could be seeking everything or fail to summon time for completion of anything

● **For realisation of potential**
Their own idea of potential is never reached despite constant striving or anxiety is such that they never get started

● **For air**
Breathes without assistance

● **For food and drink**
Able to select, provide and cook own food. May allow insufficient time for eating and drinking

● **For elimination**
May give less time for elimination. Bowel activity could be increased

● **For shelter**
May choose inappropriate clothes to wear. Could be fastidious or neglectful of caring for shelter

● **For exercise**
Always moving and involved in activity

● **For sleep/rest**
Sleeps for short periods, easily roused and consistently tired

**SELF-FULFILMENT
NEEDS**

**PHYSIOLOGICAL
NEEDS**

**11.   AN ANXIOUS PERSON,
IRRITABLE AND
HYPERACTIVE**

**ACHIEVEMENT
NEEDS**

**SECURITY NEEDS**

● **For approval**
Always seeking approval due to lack of self-confidence and time given to build up relationships

● **For respect**
Always seeking approval due to lack of self-confidence and time given to relationships

● **For maintenance of dignity**
May be easily threatened or disinterested

● **For safety at home**
Tendency to be forgetful of hazards while moving rapidly from task to task

● **For safety at school/work**
Tendency to be forgetful of hazards while moving rapidly from task to task

● **For affection**
Tendency to have a wide circle of acquaintances due to moving from group to group

● **For a sense of belonging**
Wants to belong to everything, often unrealistic in expectations

**Figure 2.13**  *An underactive person profile*

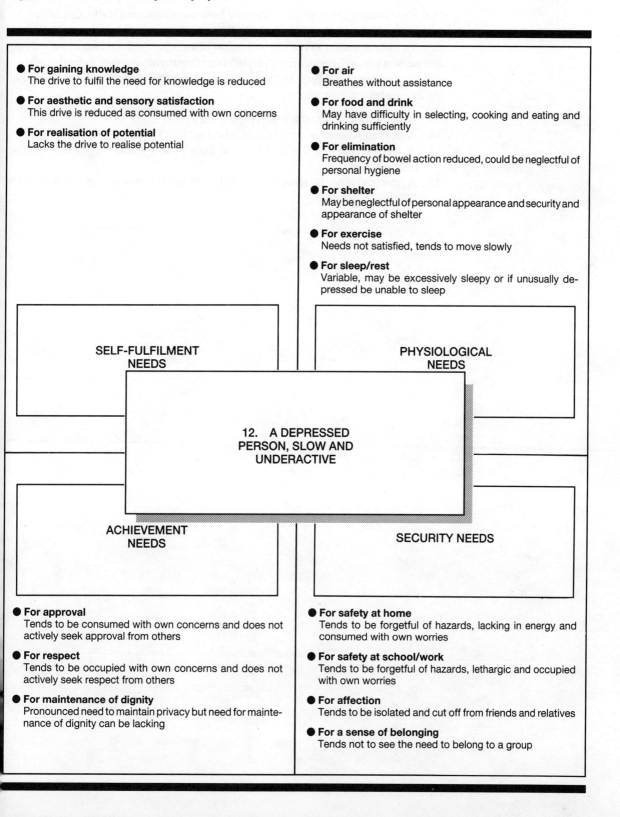

● **For gaining knowledge**
The drive to fulfil the need for knowledge is reduced

● **For aesthetic and sensory satisfaction**
This drive is reduced as consumed with own concerns

● **For realisation of potential**
Lacks the drive to realise potential

● **For air**
Breathes without assistance

● **For food and drink**
May have difficulty in selecting, cooking and eating and drinking sufficiently

● **For elimination**
Frequency of bowel action reduced, could be neglectful of personal hygiene

● **For shelter**
May be neglectful of personal appearance and security and appearance of shelter

● **For exercise**
Needs not satisfied, tends to move slowly

● **For sleep/rest**
Variable, may be excessively sleepy or if unusually depressed be unable to sleep

SELF-FULFILMENT
NEEDS

PHYSIOLOGICAL
NEEDS

12.   A DEPRESSED
PERSON, SLOW AND
UNDERACTIVE

ACHIEVEMENT
NEEDS

SECURITY NEEDS

● **For approval**
Tends to be consumed with own concerns and does not actively seek approval from others

● **For respect**
Tends to be occupied with own concerns and does not actively seek respect from others

● **For maintenance of dignity**
Pronounced need to maintain privacy but need for maintenance of dignity can be lacking

● **For safety at home**
Tends to be forgetful of hazards, lacking in energy and consumed with own worries

● **For safety at school/work**
Tends to be forgetful of hazards, lethargic and occupied with own worries

● **For affection**
Tends to be isolated and cut off from friends and relatives

● **For a sense of belonging**
Tends not to see the need to belong to a group

## EFFECTS OF SOCIAL/CULTURAL STATUS

Here are some chosen profiles to show how *social/cultural* status can affect the ways in which needs are satisfied. By social or cultural status we mean a person's place within a type of civilisation in an organised community involving the person's health, education, physical environment, income, poverty, effects of public order and safety, recreation and their participation and/or alienation. As examples we have chosen:

13. A person of no fixed abode (*Figure 2.14*).
14. A person who lives alone in an urban setting (*Figure 2.15*).
15. A person who is a member of a family unit living in a rural setting (*Figure 2.16*).
16. A person who is living in a different culture/society to his/her own (*Figure 2.17*).

**Figure 2.14**    *Profile of a person of no fixed abode*

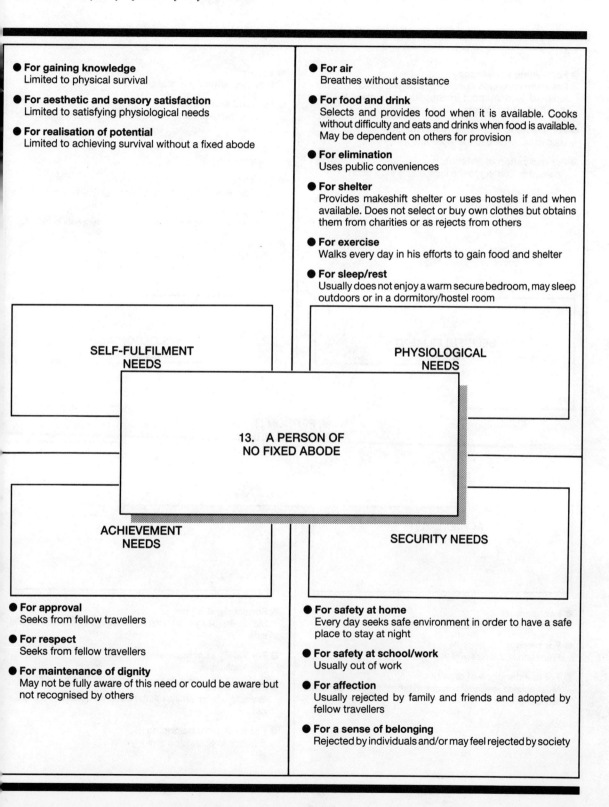

● **For gaining knowledge**
Limited to physical survival

● **For aesthetic and sensory satisfaction**
Limited to satisfying physiological needs

● **For realisation of potential**
Limited to achieving survival without a fixed abode

● **For air**
Breathes without assistance

● **For food and drink**
Selects and provides food when it is available. Cooks without difficulty and eats and drinks when food is available. May be dependent on others for provision

● **For elimination**
Uses public conveniences

● **For shelter**
Provides makeshift shelter or uses hostels if and when available. Does not select or buy own clothes but obtains them from charities or as rejects from others

● **For exercise**
Walks every day in his efforts to gain food and shelter

● **For sleep/rest**
Usually does not enjoy a warm secure bedroom, may sleep outdoors or in a dormitory/hostel room

SELF-FULFILMENT
NEEDS

PHYSIOLOGICAL
NEEDS

13.   A PERSON OF
NO FIXED ABODE

ACHIEVEMENT
NEEDS

SECURITY NEEDS

● **For approval**
Seeks from fellow travellers

● **For respect**
Seeks from fellow travellers

● **For maintenance of dignity**
May not be fully aware of this need or could be aware but not recognised by others

● **For safety at home**
Every day seeks safe environment in order to have a safe place to stay at night

● **For safety at school/work**
Usually out of work

● **For affection**
Usually rejected by family and friends and adopted by fellow travellers

● **For a sense of belonging**
Rejected by individuals and/or may feel rejected by society

**Figure 2.15**  *Profile of a person living alone*

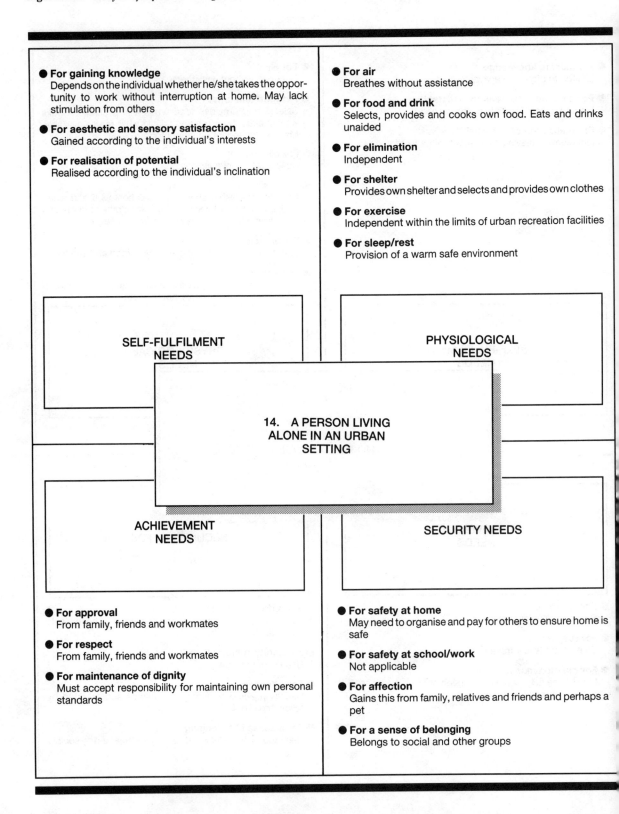

● **For gaining knowledge**
Depends on the individual whether he/she takes the opportunity to work without interruption at home. May lack
stimulation from others

● **For aesthetic and sensory satisfaction**
Gained according to the individual's interests

● **For realisation of potential**
Realised according to the individual's inclination

● **For air**
Breathes without assistance

● **For food and drink**
Selects, provides and cooks own food. Eats and drinks
unaided

● **For elimination**
Independent

● **For shelter**
Provides own shelter and selects and provides own clothes

● **For exercise**
Independent within the limits of urban recreation facilities

● **For sleep/rest**
Provision of a warm safe environment

**SELF-FULFILMENT
NEEDS**

**PHYSIOLOGICAL
NEEDS**

**14.    A PERSON LIVING
ALONE IN AN URBAN
SETTING**

**ACHIEVEMENT
NEEDS**

**SECURITY NEEDS**

● **For approval**
From family, friends and workmates

● **For respect**
From family, friends and workmates

● **For maintenance of dignity**
Must accept responsibility for maintaining own personal
standards

● **For safety at home**
May need to organise and pay for others to ensure home is
safe

● **For safety at school/work**
Not applicable

● **For affection**
Gains this from family, relatives and friends and perhaps a
pet

● **For a sense of belonging**
Belongs to social and other groups

**Figure 2.16**   *Profile of a person living in a family*

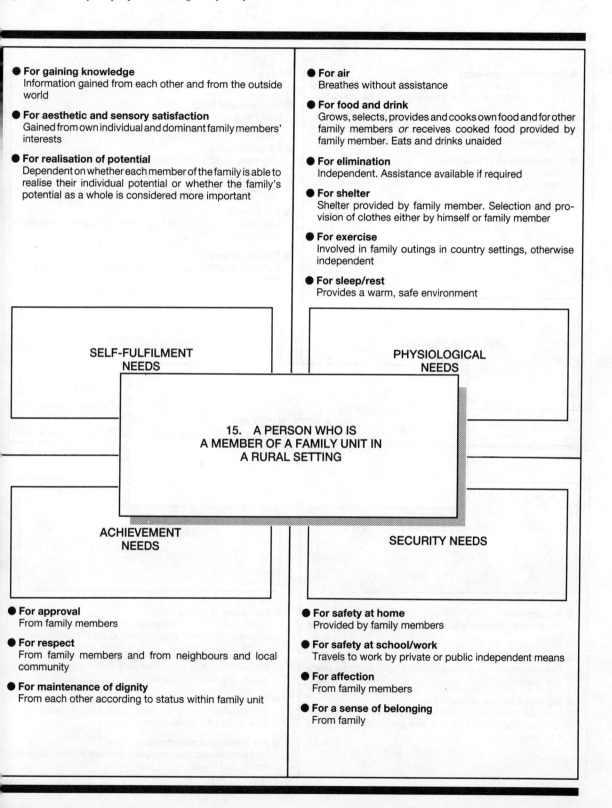

● **For gaining knowledge**
Information gained from each other and from the outside world

● **For aesthetic and sensory satisfaction**
Gained from own individual and dominant family members' interests

● **For realisation of potential**
Dependent on whether each member of the family is able to realise their individual potential or whether the family's potential as a whole is considered more important

● **For air**
Breathes without assistance

● **For food and drink**
Grows, selects, provides and cooks own food and for other family members *or* receives cooked food provided by family member. Eats and drinks unaided

● **For elimination**
Independent. Assistance available if required

● **For shelter**
Shelter provided by family member. Selection and provision of clothes either by himself or family member

● **For exercise**
Involved in family outings in country settings, otherwise independent

● **For sleep/rest**
Provides a warm, safe environment

SELF-FULFILMENT
NEEDS

PHYSIOLOGICAL
NEEDS

15.   A PERSON WHO IS
A MEMBER OF A FAMILY UNIT IN
A RURAL SETTING

ACHIEVEMENT
NEEDS

SECURITY NEEDS

● **For approval**
From family members

● **For respect**
From family members and from neighbours and local community

● **For maintenance of dignity**
From each other according to status within family unit

● **For safety at home**
Provided by family members

● **For safety at school/work**
Travels to work by private or public independent means

● **For affection**
From family members

● **For a sense of belonging**
From family

**Figure 2.17**   *Profile of a person living within a different culture / society*

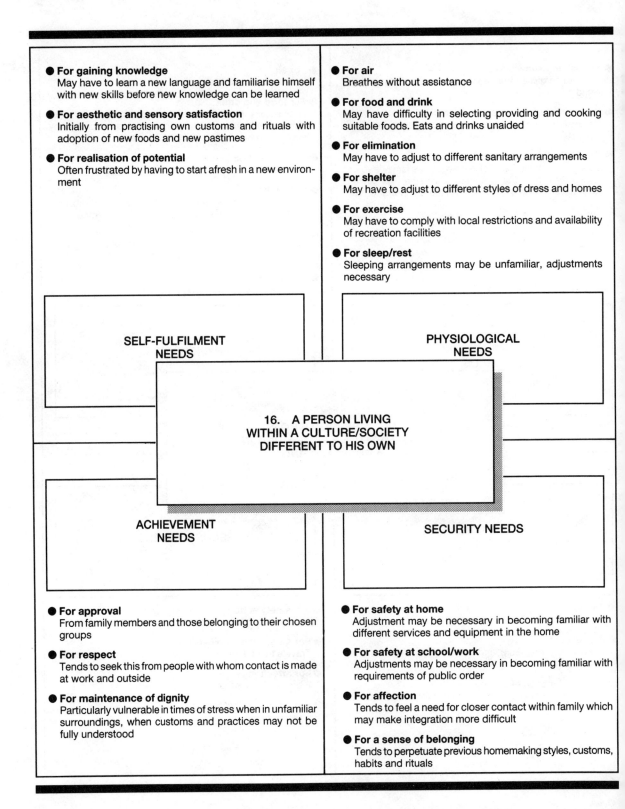

● **For gaining knowledge**
May have to learn a new language and familiarise himself with new skills before new knowledge can be learned

● **For aesthetic and sensory satisfaction**
Initially from practising own customs and rituals with adoption of new foods and new pastimes

● **For realisation of potential**
Often frustrated by having to start afresh in a new environment

● **For air**
Breathes without assistance

● **For food and drink**
May have difficulty in selecting providing and cooking suitable foods. Eats and drinks unaided

● **For elimination**
May have to adjust to different sanitary arrangements

● **For shelter**
May have to adjust to different styles of dress and homes

● **For exercise**
May have to comply with local restrictions and availability of recreation facilities

● **For sleep/rest**
Sleeping arrangements may be unfamiliar, adjustments necessary

SELF-FULFILMENT
NEEDS

PHYSIOLOGICAL
NEEDS

16.   A PERSON LIVING
WITHIN A CULTURE/SOCIETY
DIFFERENT TO HIS OWN

ACHIEVEMENT
NEEDS

SECURITY NEEDS

● **For approval**
From family members and those belonging to their chosen groups

● **For respect**
Tends to seek this from people with whom contact is made at work and outside

● **For maintenance of dignity**
Particularly vulnerable in times of stress when in unfamiliar surroundings, when customs and practices may not be fully understood

● **For safety at home**
Adjustment may be necessary in becoming familiar with different services and equipment in the home

● **For safety at school/work**
Adjustments may be necessary in becoming familiar with requirements of public order

● **For affection**
Tends to feel a need for closer contact within family which may make integration more difficult

● **For a sense of belonging**
Tends to perpetuate previous homemaking styles, customs, habits and rituals

## EFFECTS OF PHYSICAL AND INTELLECTUAL CAPACITY

Here are some chosen profiles to show how *physical and intellectual capacity* can affect the ways in which needs are satisfied. It is accepted as normal that an individual can move, see, hear and be within acceptable limits for body weight and height and intelligence. These factors are illustrated on the left of *Table 2.1*. The changes in physical and intellectual capacity are listed on the right and the numbers 17 to 22 refer to the profiles illustrated in *Figures 2.17* to *2.22*.

Table 2.1   *Chart to illustrate normal and abnormal physical and intellectual capacities*

| **Physical capacity**<br>Normal weight and height for age and sex | 17. Overweight and underweight |
|---|---|
| Normal mobility | 18. Loss of mobility |
| Able to see | 19. Loss of sight |
| Able to hear | 20. Loss of hearing |
| **Intellectual capacity**<br>Intelligence quotient around 100 | 21. High intelligence quotient (gifted)<br><br>22. Low intelligence quotient (educationally subnormal) |

**Figure 2.18**   *Profile of a person who is at the limits of normal height and weight*

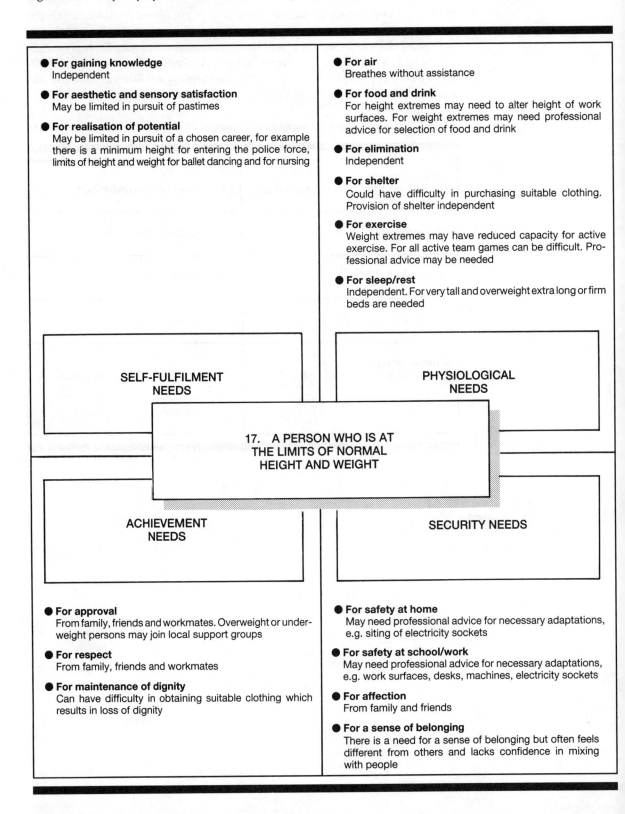

● **For gaining knowledge**
Independent

● **For aesthetic and sensory satisfaction**
May be limited in pursuit of pastimes

● **For realisation of potential**
May be limited in pursuit of a chosen career, for example there is a minimum height for entering the police force, limits of height and weight for ballet dancing and for nursing

● **For air**
Breathes without assistance

● **For food and drink**
For height extremes may need to alter height of work surfaces. For weight extremes may need professional advice for selection of food and drink

● **For elimination**
Independent

● **For shelter**
Could have difficulty in purchasing suitable clothing. Provision of shelter independent

● **For exercise**
Weight extremes may have reduced capacity for active exercise. For all active team games can be difficult. Professional advice may be needed

● **For sleep/rest**
Independent. For very tall and overweight extra long or firm beds are needed

**SELF-FULFILMENT NEEDS**

**PHYSIOLOGICAL NEEDS**

**17.   A PERSON WHO IS AT THE LIMITS OF NORMAL HEIGHT AND WEIGHT**

**ACHIEVEMENT NEEDS**

**SECURITY NEEDS**

● **For approval**
From family, friends and workmates. Overweight or underweight persons may join local support groups

● **For respect**
From family, friends and workmates

● **For maintenance of dignity**
Can have difficulty in obtaining suitable clothing which results in loss of dignity

● **For safety at home**
May need professional advice for necessary adaptations, e.g. siting of electricity sockets

● **For safety at school/work**
May need professional advice for necessary adaptations, e.g. work surfaces, desks, machines, electricity sockets

● **For affection**
From family and friends

● **For a sense of belonging**
There is a need for a sense of belonging but often feels different from others and lacks confidence in mixing with people

**Figure 2.19** *Profile of a person with loss of mobility*

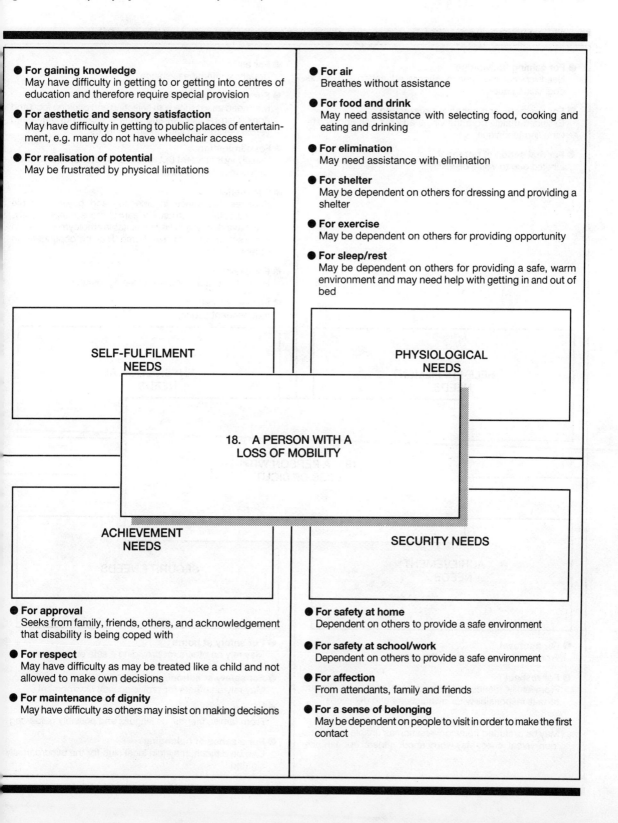

● **For gaining knowledge**
May have difficulty in getting to or getting into centres of education and therefore require special provision

● **For aesthetic and sensory satisfaction**
May have difficulty in getting to public places of entertainment, e.g. many do not have wheelchair access

● **For realisation of potential**
May be frustrated by physical limitations

● **For air**
Breathes without assistance

● **For food and drink**
May need assistance with selecting food, cooking and eating and drinking

● **For elimination**
May need assistance with elimination

● **For shelter**
May be dependent on others for dressing and providing a shelter

● **For exercise**
May be dependent on others for providing opportunity

● **For sleep/rest**
May be dependent on others for providing a safe, warm environment and may need help with getting in and out of bed

**SELF-FULFILMENT
NEEDS**

**PHYSIOLOGICAL
NEEDS**

**18.  A PERSON WITH A
LOSS OF MOBILITY**

**ACHIEVEMENT
NEEDS**

**SECURITY NEEDS**

● **For approval**
Seeks from family, friends, others, and acknowledgement that disability is being coped with

● **For respect**
May have difficulty as may be treated like a child and not allowed to make own decisions

● **For maintenance of dignity**
May have difficulty as others may insist on making decisions

● **For safety at home**
Dependent on others to provide a safe environment

● **For safety at school/work**
Dependent on others to provide a safe environment

● **For affection**
From attendants, family and friends

● **For a sense of belonging**
May be dependent on people to visit in order to make the first contact

**Figure 2.20**   *Profile of a person with loss of sight*

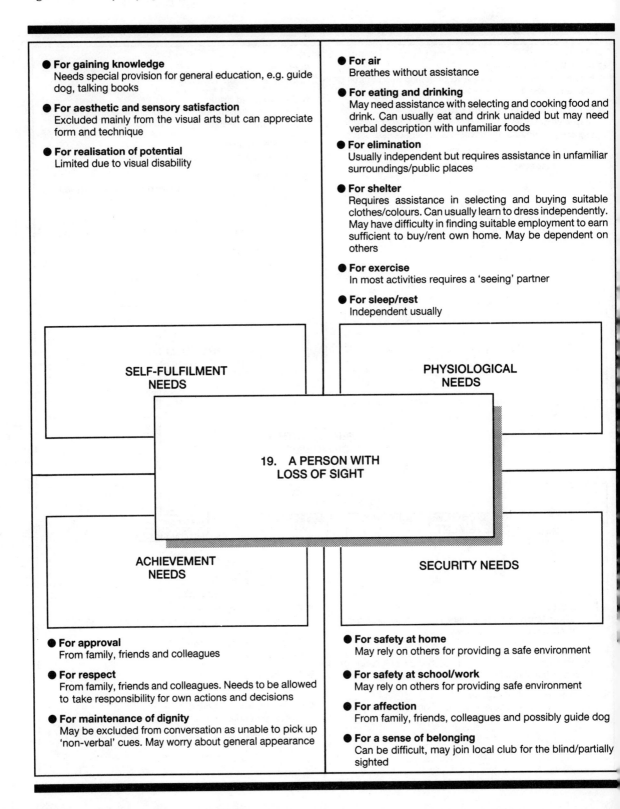

● **For gaining knowledge**
Needs special provision for general education, e.g. guide dog, talking books

● **For aesthetic and sensory satisfaction**
Excluded mainly from the visual arts but can appreciate form and technique

● **For realisation of potential**
Limited due to visual disability

● **For air**
Breathes without assistance

● **For eating and drinking**
May need assistance with selecting and cooking food and drink. Can usually eat and drink unaided but may need verbal description with unfamiliar foods

● **For elimination**
Usually independent but requires assistance in unfamiliar surroundings/public places

● **For shelter**
Requires assistance in selecting and buying suitable clothes/colours. Can usually learn to dress independently. May have difficulty in finding suitable employment to earn sufficient to buy/rent own home. May be dependent on others

● **For exercise**
In most activities requires a 'seeing' partner

● **For sleep/rest**
Independent usually

**SELF-FULFILMENT NEEDS**

**PHYSIOLOGICAL NEEDS**

**19.   A PERSON WITH LOSS OF SIGHT**

**ACHIEVEMENT NEEDS**

**SECURITY NEEDS**

● **For approval**
From family, friends and colleagues

● **For respect**
From family, friends and colleagues. Needs to be allowed to take responsibility for own actions and decisions

● **For maintenance of dignity**
May be excluded from conversation as unable to pick up 'non-verbal' cues. May worry about general appearance

● **For safety at home**
May rely on others for providing a safe environment

● **For safety at school/work**
May rely on others for providing safe environment

● **For affection**
From family, friends, colleagues and possibly guide dog

● **For a sense of belonging**
Can be difficult, may join local club for the blind/partially sighted

**Figure 2.21**   *Profile of a person with loss of hearing*

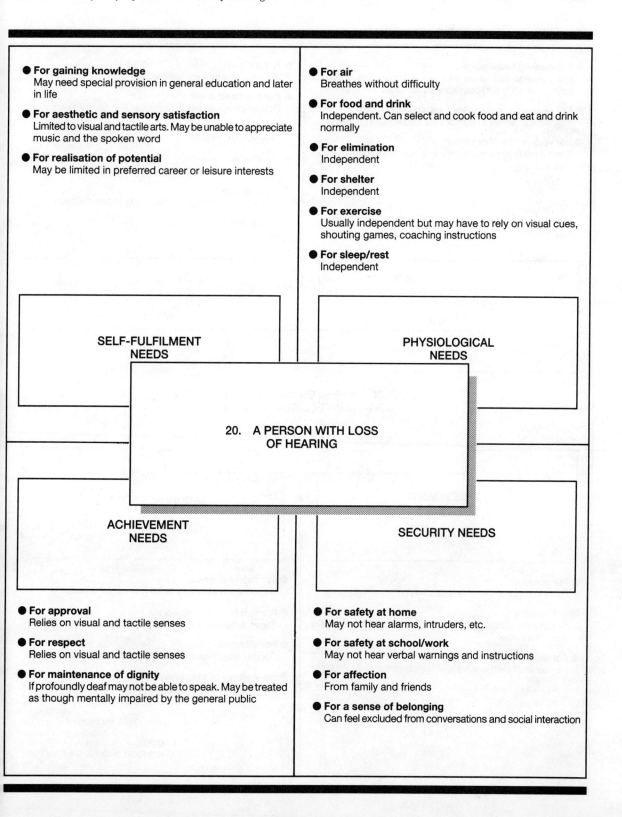

● **For gaining knowledge**
May need special provision in general education and later in life

● **For aesthetic and sensory satisfaction**
Limited to visual and tactile arts. May be unable to appreciate music and the spoken word

● **For realisation of potential**
May be limited in preferred career or leisure interests

● **For air**
Breathes without difficulty

● **For food and drink**
Independent. Can select and cook food and eat and drink normally

● **For elimination**
Independent

● **For shelter**
Independent

● **For exercise**
Usually independent but may have to rely on visual cues, shouting games, coaching instructions

● **For sleep/rest**
Independent

**SELF-FULFILMENT NEEDS**

**PHYSIOLOGICAL NEEDS**

**20.   A PERSON WITH LOSS OF HEARING**

**ACHIEVEMENT NEEDS**

**SECURITY NEEDS**

● **For approval**
Relies on visual and tactile senses

● **For respect**
Relies on visual and tactile senses

● **For maintenance of dignity**
If profoundly deaf may not be able to speak. May be treated as though mentally impaired by the general public

● **For safety at home**
May not hear alarms, intruders, etc.

● **For safety at school/work**
May not hear verbal warnings and instructions

● **For affection**
From family and friends

● **For a sense of belonging**
Can feel excluded from conversations and social interaction

**Figure 2.22**  *Profile of a person with above average intelligence*

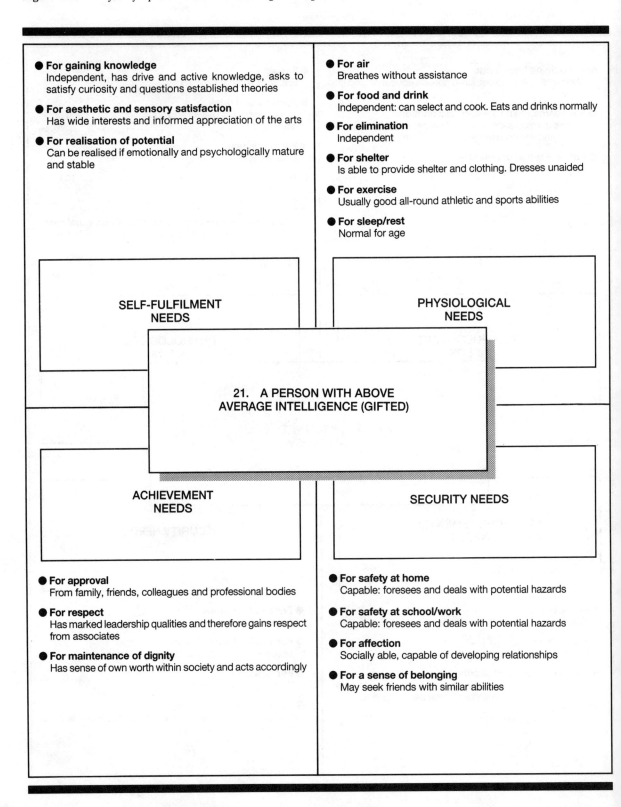

● **For gaining knowledge**
Independent, has drive and active knowledge, asks to satisfy curiosity and questions established theories

● **For aesthetic and sensory satisfaction**
Has wide interests and informed appreciation of the arts

● **For realisation of potential**
Can be realised if emotionally and psychologically mature and stable

● **For air**
Breathes without assistance

● **For food and drink**
Independent: can select and cook. Eats and drinks normally

● **For elimination**
Independent

● **For shelter**
Is able to provide shelter and clothing. Dresses unaided

● **For exercise**
Usually good all-round athletic and sports abilities

● **For sleep/rest**
Normal for age

SELF-FULFILMENT
NEEDS

PHYSIOLOGICAL
NEEDS

21.   A PERSON WITH ABOVE
AVERAGE INTELLIGENCE (GIFTED)

ACHIEVEMENT
NEEDS

SECURITY NEEDS

● **For approval**
From family, friends, colleagues and professional bodies

● **For respect**
Has marked leadership qualities and therefore gains respect from associates

● **For maintenance of dignity**
Has sense of own worth within society and acts accordingly

● **For safety at home**
Capable: foresees and deals with potential hazards

● **For safety at school/work**
Capable: foresees and deals with potential hazards

● **For affection**
Socially able, capable of developing relationships

● **For a sense of belonging**
May seek friends with similar abilities

**Figure 2.23**    *Profile of a person with low intelligence*

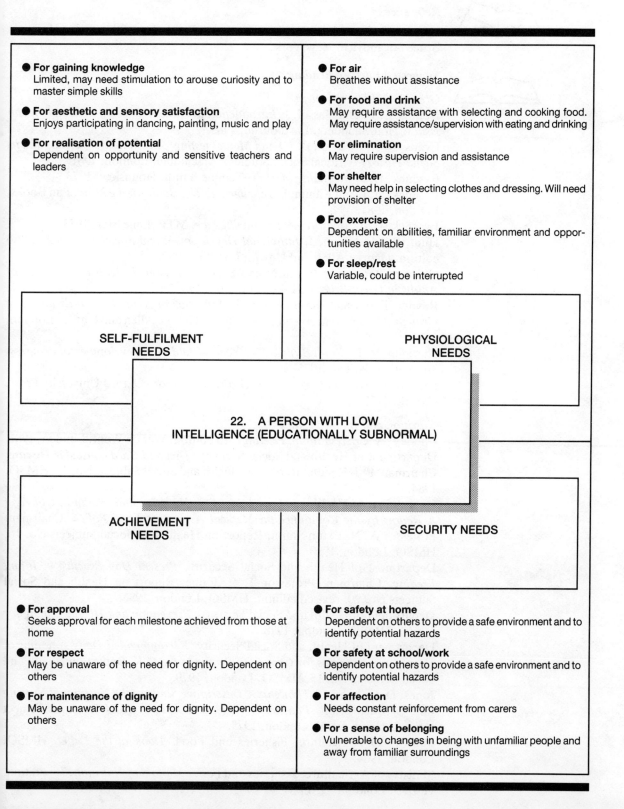

● **For gaining knowledge**
Limited, may need stimulation to arouse curiosity and to master simple skills

● **For aesthetic and sensory satisfaction**
Enjoys participating in dancing, painting, music and play

● **For realisation of potential**
Dependent on opportunity and sensitive teachers and leaders

● **For air**
Breathes without assistance

● **For food and drink**
May require assistance with selecting and cooking food. May require assistance/supervision with eating and drinking

● **For elimination**
May require supervision and assistance

● **For shelter**
May need help in selecting clothes and dressing. Will need provision of shelter

● **For exercise**
Dependent on abilities, familiar environment and opportunities available

● **For sleep/rest**
Variable, could be interrupted

SELF-FULFILMENT
NEEDS

PHYSIOLOGICAL
NEEDS

22.   A PERSON WITH LOW
INTELLIGENCE (EDUCATIONALLY SUBNORMAL)

ACHIEVEMENT
NEEDS

SECURITY NEEDS

● **For approval**
Seeks approval for each milestone achieved from those at home

● **For respect**
May be unaware of the need for dignity. Dependent on others

● **For maintenance of dignity**
May be unaware of the need for dignity. Dependent on others

● **For safety at home**
Dependent on others to provide a safe environment and to identify potential hazards

● **For safety at school/work**
Dependent on others to provide a safe environment and to identify potential hazards

● **For affection**
Needs constant reinforcement from carers

● **For a sense of belonging**
Vulnerable to changes in being with unfamiliar people and away from familiar surroundings

## REFERENCES AND FURTHER READING

### Reference

Hilgard, E. R. *et al.* (1983). *Introduction to Psychology,* 8th edition. Harcourt Bruce Jovanovich, New York.

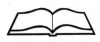

### *Suggested Further Reading*

*Growth and Development*

Dennis, L. B. and Hassol, J. *Introduction to Human Development and Health Issues.* Holt-Saunders, Eastbourne, 1983.

Evans, B. and Waites, B. *IQ and Mental testing: An Unnatural Science and its Social History* (Critical Social Studies). Macmillan, London, 1981.

Eysenck, H. J. *Inequality of Man.* Temple Smith, Hounslow, 1973.

Eysenck, H. J. and Kamin, L. *Intelligence: The Battle for the Mind.* Pan Books, London, 1981.

Eysenck, H. J. *Measurement of Intelligence.* MTP, Lancaster, 1973.

Hunt, S. and Hilton, J. *Individual Development and Social Experience*, 2nd edition. George Allen and Unwin, London, 1981.

Office of Population Censuses and Survey Division. *Heights and Weights of Adults in Great Britain.* HMSO, London, 1984.

Rayner, E. *Human Development: An Introduction to the Psycho-dynamics of Growth, Maturity and Ageing*, 2nd edition. George Allen and Unwin, London, 1978.

Sheridan, M. D. *From Birth to Five Years: Children's Developmental Progress*, 3rd edition. NFER, 1975.

Sinclair, D. *Human Growth after Birth*, 3rd edition. Oxford University Press, Oxford, 1978.

*Nutrition and Infant Feeding*

Chetley, A. *Crisis in Infant Feeding*, 3rd edition. War on Want, London, 1981.

Department of Health and Social Security. *Diet and Cardiovascular Disease.* Chairman: P. J. Rendle. Report on Health and Social Subjects No. 28, HMSO, 1984.

Department of Health and Social Security. *Nutrition and Health in Old Age: A Report by the Committee on Medical Aspects of Food Policy.* Chairman: Professor A. N. Exton-Smith. Report on Health and Social Subjects No. 16, HMSO, London, 1980.

Department of Health and Social Security. *Present Day Practice in Infant Feeding.* Chairman: Professor T. E. Oppe. Report on Health and Social Subjects No. 20, revised edition, HMSO, London, 1983.

Department of Health and Social Security. *Prevention and Health: Eating for Health.* HMSO, London, 1978.

Department of Health and Social Security. *Recommended Daily Amounts of Energy and Nutrients for Groups of People in the U.K.* Report on Health and Social Subjects No. 15, HMSO, London, 1979.

Jones, D. C. *Food for Thought: A Descriptive Study of the Nutritional Nursing Care of Unconscious Patients in General Hospitals.* RCN Research Project series 2, No. 4, RCN, London, 1975.

Ministry of Agriculture, Fisheries and Food. *Look at the Label.* HMSO, London, 1984.

Ministry of Agriculture, Fisheries and Food. *Manual of Nutrition*, 7th edition. HMSO, London, 1970.

National Advisory Committee on Nutrition Education. *Proposal for Nutritional Guidelines for Health Education in Britain.* Chairman: Professor U.P.T. James. Health Education Council, London, 1983.

Parsonage, S. and Clark, J. *Infant Feeding and Family Nutrition* (Topics in Community Health). HM&M Publications, Chichester, 1981.

Scowen, P. and Wells, J. *Feeding Children in the First Year.* Health Visitor's Association, London, 1979.

*Immunisation*

Department of Health and Social Security, Scottish Home and Health Department. *Immunisation Against Infectious Disease.* HMSO, London, 1982.

Department of Health and Social Security. *Whooping Cough: Reports from the Committee on Safety of Medicines and the Joint Committee on Vaccination and Immunisation.* Chairman: Professor A. Goldberg. HMSO, London, 1981.

Dick, G. *Immunisation.* Update Publications, London, 1978.

Illingworth, R. S. *Infections and Immunisation of Your Child.* Patient Handbook No. 6, Churchill Livingstone, Edinburgh, 1981.

Office of Health Economics. *Childhood Vaccination: Current Controversies* (Current Health Problems No. 76). OHE, London, 1984.

Royal College of Nursing. *Guidelines on Immunisations.* RCN, London, 1977.

*Social Welfare and Social History*

Abel-Smith, B. *National Health Service: The First Thirty Years.* HMSO, London, 1978.

Baly, M. E. *Nursing and Social Change*, 2nd edition. Heinemann, London, 1980.

Brechin, A. *et al. Handicap in a Social World.* Hodder and Stoughton, London, 1981.

Crombie, D. L. *Social Class and Health Status: Inequality or Difference.* Royal College of General Practitioners, Exeter, 1984.

Davies, B. M. *Community Health and Social Services*, 4th edition. Hodder and Stoughton, London, 1984.

Department of Health and Social Security. *Inequalities in Health: Report of a Research Working Group.* DHSS, London, 1980.

Gaffin, J. (Ed.). *Nurse and the Welfare State* (Topics in Community Health). HM&M, Chichester, 1981.

Ham, C. *Health Policy in Britain: The Politics and Organisation of the National Health Service.* Macmillan, London, 1982.

Mooney, G. H. *et al. Choices for Health Care.* Macmillan, London, 1980.

Sticker, P. *Stigma and Social Welfare.* Croom Helm, Beckenham, 1984.

Townsend, P. *Poverty in the United Kingdom: A Survey of Household Resources and Standards of Living.* Penguin Books, Harmondsworth, Middx. 1980.

Walters, V. *Class Inequality and Health Care: The Origins and Impact of the National Health Service.* Croom Helm, Beckenham, 1980.

Watkin, B. *The National Health Service: The First Phase 1948–1974 and After.* Allen and Unwin, London, 1978.

*Ethnic Minorities and Support*

Age Concern. *Black and Asian Old People in Britain: First Report of a Research Study* (Research perspectives on ageing). Age Concern, Mitcham, 1984.

Health Education Council and National Extension College for Training in Health and Race. *Providing Effective Health Care in a Multiracial Society.*

Health Education Council, London, 1984.

Henley, A. (Asians in Britain Series):

1. *Caring for Muslims and their Families: Religious Aspects of Care*, 1982.
2. *Caring for Hindus and their Families: Religious Aspects of Care*, 1983.
3. *Caring for Sikhs and their Families: Religious Aspects of Care*, 1983.

Published by the DHSS and King's Fund Centre.

Hughes, J. *et al.* (Eds). *Race and Employment in the NHS*. King's Fund Centre, London, 1984.

Lothian Community Relations Council. *Religions and Cultures: A Guide to Patients' Beliefs for Health Service Staff*, 2nd edition. Loth. Comm. Rel. Council, Lothian, 1984.

McDermott, M. Y. and Ahsan, M. M. *Muslim Guide for Teachers, Employers, Community and Social administrators in Britain*. Islamic Foundation, Leicester, 1980.

Rack, P. *Race, Culture and Mental Disorder*. Tavistock Publications, London, 1982.

Sampson, A. C. M. *The Neglected Ethic: Cultural and Religious Factors in Care of Patients*. McGraw-Hill, Maidenhead, 1982.

*Journal*

*Health and Race*. Quarterly Newsletter produced by Training in Health and Race, Leeds CVS, Leeds.

*Ageing*

Aiken, L. *Later life*. Holt-Saunders, Eastbourne, 1978.

Blythe, R. *View in Winter: Reflections in Old Age*. Viking, London, 1979.

Bromley, D. B. *Psychology of Human Ageing*, 2nd edition. Penguin Books, Harmondsworth, Middx, 1974.

Coni, N. *et al. Ageing: the Facts*. Oxford University Press, Oxford, 1984.

Garrett, G. *Health Needs of the Elderly*. Essentials of Nursing Series, Macmillan, London, 1983.

Gray, M. and Wilcock, G. *Our Elders*. Oxford University Press, Oxford, 1981.

Hobman, D. (Ed.). *Impact of Ageing*. Croom Helm, Beckenham, 1981.

Pincus, L. *Challenge of a Long life*. Faber and Faber, London, 1981.

Shaw, M. W. *Challenge of Ageing: A Multidisciplinary Approach to Extended Care*. Churchill Livingstone, Edinburgh, 1984.

*Accommodation For, and Care Of, the Elderly*

Age Concern. *Housing for Ethnic Elders*. Age Concern Publications, Mitcham 1984.

Beth Johnson Foundation. *Quality of Life of the Elderly in Residential Homes and Hospitals*. BJF, 1977.

Centre for Policy on Ageing. *Home Life: A Code of Practice for Residential Care, a Report of a Working Party*. Chairman: Lady Avebury. CPA, London 1984.

Norman, A. *Bricks and Mortals: Design and Lifestyles in Old People's Homes* CPA, London, 1984.

Shaw, M. W. *Challenge of Ageing: A Multidisciplinary Approach to Extended Care*. Churchill Livingstone, Edinburgh, 1984.

Wade, B. *et al. Dependency with Dignity: Different Care Provisions for the Elderly*. Occupational papers on Social Administration. National Council for Voluntary Organisations, London, 1983.

# Section 2   The Patient

## Introduction

We have looked at need fulfilment for various groups of individuals and we look now in detail at individuals who have superimposed pathology. For each of the first four chapters in this section one of the living activities, i.e. Breathing, Eating and Drinking, Eliminating and Sleeping and Resting, is identified and then considered using the following headings in turn.

● References for revision of associated normal physiology.
● Sociological factors affecting the activity.
● Psychological factors affecting the activity.
● A patient history.
● Explanation of clinical features.
● Effects of failure of identified living activity on other activities.
● A method to assist you in assessing the chosen patient.
● Choosing nursing actions to assist the chosen patient with difficulty in living activities.
● Explanation for choice of nursing actions.
● Choosing priorities in nursing actions.
● Identification of criteria for progress.
● Identification of long-term goals.

At the end of each chapter you will find a selection of further medical and surgical conditions which may affect living activities, with suggested further reading of selected aspects of pharmacology, physiotherapy and nursing procedures and techniques.

For Chapter 7 we have chosen a patient who has difficulty with moving and we show how all the living activities can be affected in the one study. This study is preceded by a series of information sheets for each of the remaining living activities.

# Chapter 3
# Breathing

## NORMAL PHYSIOLOGY

Before proceeding we suggest you revise your knowledge of normal physiology of breathing by using the following references (given in full in *References*) or any other suitable textbook:

- Hunt and Sendell (1987). *Nursing the Adult with a Specific Physiological Disturbance*, 2nd edn.
- Green (1978). *Basic Clinical Physiology*, pages 2–52 and 53–67.

## SOCIOLOGICAL FACTORS AFFECTING BREATHING

Breathing is affected by the environment we live in and the status position and health of individuals in society (at home and at work). The air we breathe can be polluted by dust from factory chimneys, household fires, exhaust fumes from combustion engines and cigarette, cigar and pipe smoke. Society has produced legislation to limit air pollution such as The Clean Air Acts (1956 and 1968) and has tried to influence the population through Health Education. High levels of air pollution and/or prolonged exposure to a polluted atmosphere can cause breathing difficulties and eventually lung diseases.

Some members of society may be more susceptible to breathing difficulties because of age (i.e. the young and the old), nutritional state and general state of health.

If we measure air pollution on a scale 1–10, with 1 being the cleanest air and 10 being the most polluted air, and also grade the vulnerability of an individual from 1–10, with 1 being the least vulnerable (the healthiest) and 10 being the most vulnerable (unhealthy), we can use the chart shown in *Figure 3.1* to illustrate how both the atmosphere and the vulnerability of the individual can affect breathing.

**Figure 3.1** *Chart illustrating interrelationships of the atmosphere and vulnerability of the individual*

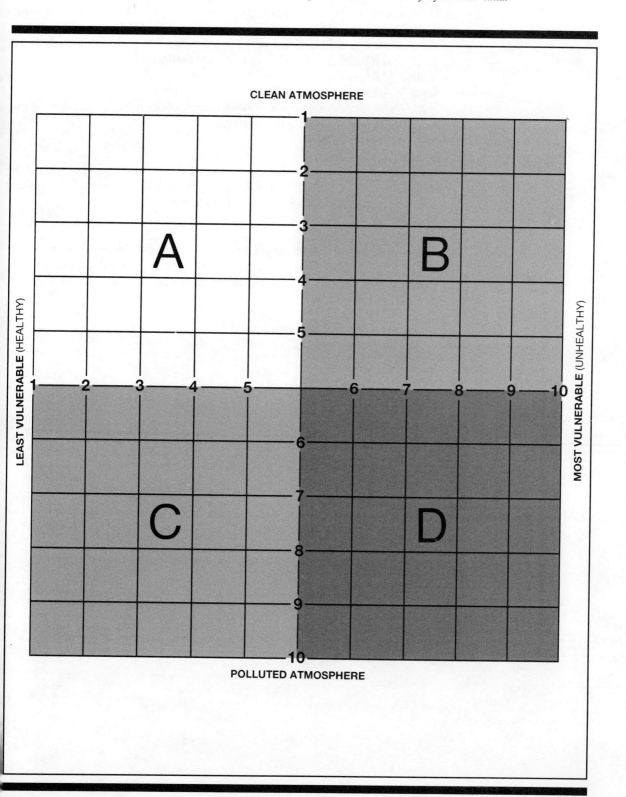

**Interrelationship of Atmospheric Pollution and the Vulnerability of the Individual**

Using the chart (*Figure 3.1*) as a graph, insert an 'X' using the two scales from the following examples.

*Mr Clarke* is a fit and active businessman who works in a modern air-conditioned office block and lives in a rural setting.

Scale 2  Vulnerability

Scale 3  Atmosphere

*Mr Jones*, a heavy smoker, works for a demolition firm. He occasionally gets a bout of bronchitis during the winter.

Scale 4  Vulnerability

Scale 9  Atmosphere

*Mr Arnold* is a retired textile worker and is now living in a heavily industrialised suburb of the city. He has chronic bronchitis and heart failure which severely restrict his mobility and independence.

Scale 9  Vulnerability

Scale 9  Atmosphere

*Mrs Simmons* has had anaemia due to lack of iron in her diet but is now recovering. She has been breathless due to the reduced oxygen-carrying capacity of the blood. She lives at the top of a steep hill in a small market town.

Scale 7  Vulnerability

Scale 3  Atmosphere

This is how your chart should look.

**Figure 3.2**    *Completed chart to illustrate the interrelationship of the atmosphere and the vulnerability of the individual*

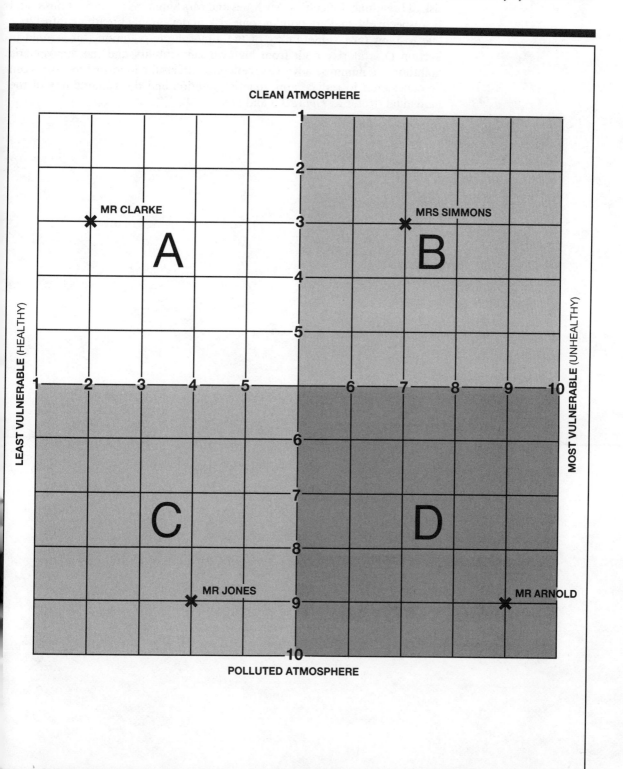

You can now see that Mr Clarke is in Section A. This section illustrates minimal risk of breathing difficulties. Mr Jones and Mrs Simmons are in Sections C and B, respectively, and are both at some risk of developing breathing difficulties due to their own vulnerability of the atmospheric pollution. Mr Arnold in Section D is at risk both from his own vulnerability and the atmospheric pollution. To minimise adverse sociological effects the following measures can be considered to reduce atmospheric pollution and the vulnerability of the individual. Refer to *Figure 3.3* and *Figure 3.4*.

**Figure 3.3**   *Factors which help to reduce atmospheric pollution*

**Legislation**

Clean Air Act (1956 and 1968)

For the reduction of atmospheric pollution in each area to deal with:

- Smoke, dust and grit pollution
- Preventive structural work by requesting prior approval for introduction of new industrial furnaces and control of chimney heights
- Introduction of smoke control areas to deal with domestic smoke pollution

**Pressure groups**

For example:

ASH:
Action on Smoking and Health

**REDUCE ATMOSPHERIC POLLUTION**

**Government circulars**

NHS Health Circular H.C.(77) 3

Non-smoking in health premises

**Health and Safety Provision**

Working conditions

Health and Safety at Work Act (1974)

**Research**

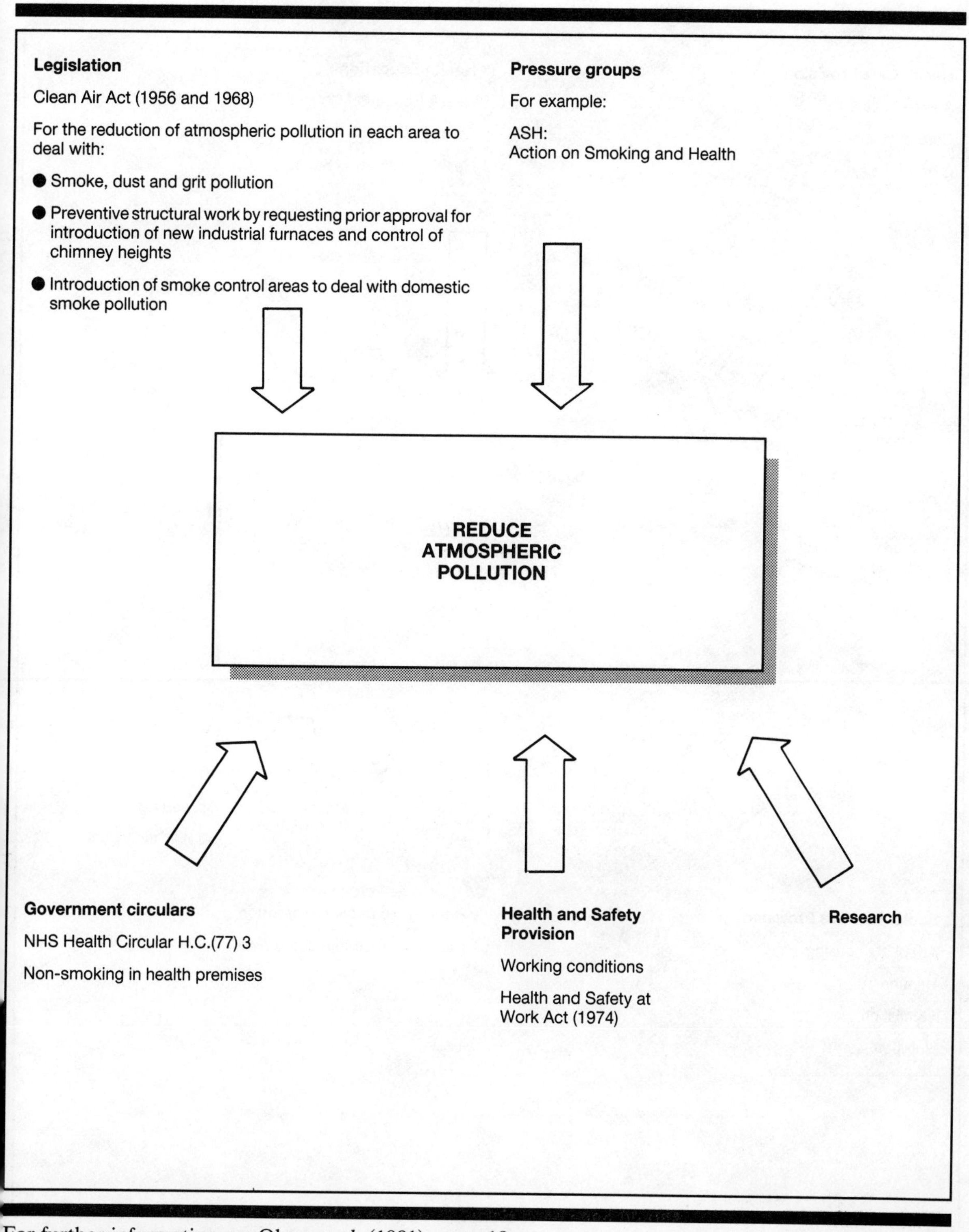

For further information see Olsen *et al.* (1981), page 18.

**Figure 3.4**    *Factors which help to reduce the vulnerability of the individual*

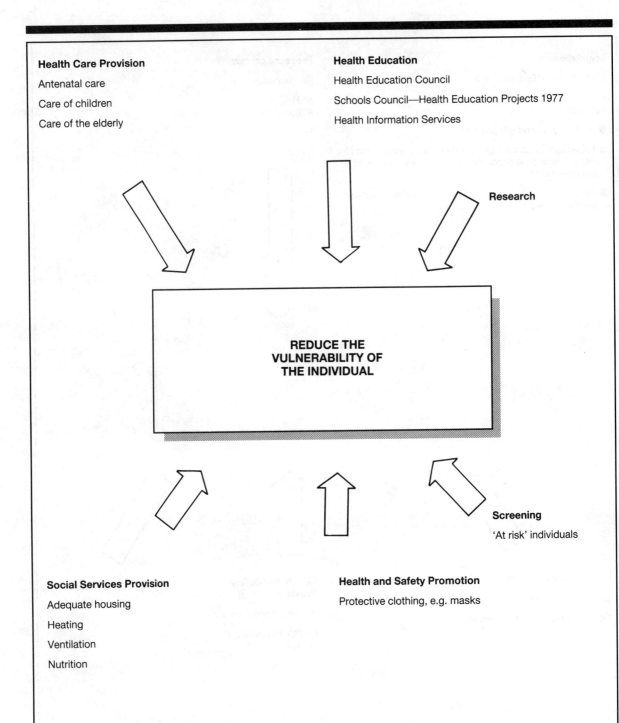

It is therefore a joint responsibility between the individual and the society he lives in to reduce risk and provide protection.

## PSYCHOLOGICAL FACTORS AFFECTING BREATHING

Psychological factors (*Figure 3.5*) can also affect breathing by causing alterations in the rate and depth of respirations by emotion, excitement, fear and anxiety.

**Figure 3.5**  *Some psychological factors affecting breathing*

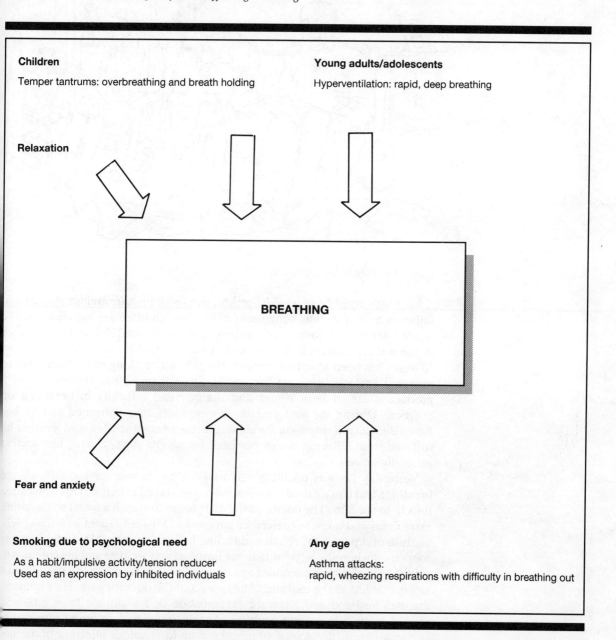

For further information see Ashton and Stepney (1982).

**PATIENT HISTORY**

Now we shall consider a patient who has difficulty in breathing. While you are reading Mr Jones' history, it is important to bear in mind the effects of air pollution and the vulnerability of Mr Jones. The clinical features of the disease affecting Mr Jones' respiratory system are explained in *Table 3.1*. See also Hunt and Sendell (1987).

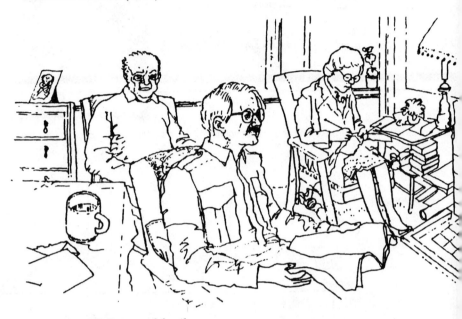

**Figure 3.6**  *Mr Jones and family*

Mr Jones, aged 58 years (*Figure 3.6*), lives with his wife and his 80-year-old father in a small mining community. Their two children are married and live nearby. Mr Jones enjoys going regularly to the local social club and is a member of the miners' choir. He has worked in the mine all his life and for the past 10 years has been a surface worker. He gave up smoking at that time due to repeated episodes of acute bronchitis. Since then he has complained of a productive cough both winter and summer and difficulty in breathing on exertion. During the past year these symptoms have worsened and he has found difficulty in singing in the choir. During a recent spell of cold weather he suffered from influenza which persisted for several days, leaving him feeling generally unwell.

Yesterday he was unable to go to work as he was having difficulty in breathing and had a raised temperature, so he stayed in bed and his wife called the GP to see him. The doctor advised Mr Jones to stay in a warm room, drink extra fluids and take the prescribed antibiotics. Mr Jones spent a restless night because of a persistent cough and feeling hot and sweaty. Mrs Jones became concerned when she noticed that her husband was weaker and his colour was greyish. He also became rather agitated and aggressive when she tried to give him his tablets in the morning. She contacted the doctor again. He explained that her husband had an acute exacerbation of his chronic bronchitis and needed to be admitted to hospital. As Mr Jones was suffering respiratory embarrassment, the doctor administered an intravenous injection of aminophylline prior to his transfer to hospital by ambulance.

*Table 3.1   Explanation of clinical features*

| Normal physiology | Abnormal physiology | Clinical features |
|---|---|---|
| (a) Air passages lined with ciliated epithelium to trap and waft debris away from the lungs up to the pharynx. | Ciliated epithelium damaged due to repeated episodes of acute bronchitis, atmospheric pollution and cold air entry, resulting in colonisation by pathogenic organisms. | Pyrexia, sweating, increased pulse rate. |
| (b) Goblet cells in the epithelium produce clear mucus to trap particles and to warm and moisten air entering the lungs. | Long-term irritation due to inhalation of coal dust results in proliferation of goblet cells and excessive manufacture of mucus. Pathogenic organisms cause the mucus to alter in consistency and colour. | Productive cough with thick, yellowish-green, offensive-smelling sputum. |
| (c) Alveoli provide a large surface area for the exchange of gases between inspired air and blood. <br><br> (d) Arterial blood gas partial pressures: <br> $PaO_2$   100 mmHg (13.5 kPa) <br> $PaCO_2$   40 mmHg (5 kPa) | Alveoli progressively destroyed leading to emphysema and reduced surface area for exchange of gases. <br><br> $PaO_2$   reduced <br> $PaCO_2$   raised | Breathlessness at rest. |
| (e) Tissues and organs require adequate oxygen perfusion to maintain function. | Inadequate perfusion of oxygen and an increase in amount of reduced haemoglobin. | Skin loses normal pink colour and becomes cyanosed. Lack of oxygen to brain results in cerebral confusion and disorientation. |
| (f) Respiration is dependent on chemical and nervous sensitivity to oxygen and carbon dioxide arterial blood levels. | Reduced sensitivity and a raised carbon dioxide arterial blood level results in respiration depending on a reduced oxygen arterial blood level, i.e. the anoxic drive. | |

## EFFECTS OF DIFFICULTY OF BREATHING ON LIVING ACTIVITIES

Breathing is normally quiet, unobtrusive and below the level of consciousness. It ensures an adequate supply of oxygen to the body tissues and the excretion of the waste products of metabolism such as carbon dioxide and water. It permits the individual to meet physiological, security, achievement and self-fulfilment needs. If a person has difficulty in breathing due to injury or disease, all the living activities can be affected as described below.

### Breathing with Difficulty

1. *Breathing*
   Noisy, obtrusive, with effort, cough (productive/non-productive).

2. *Eating and Drinking*
   Difficult to swallow when respirations rapid. Anorexia and tendency to dehydration.

3. *Eliminating*
   Poor muscle tone in bowel evacuation; lack of bulk in diet. Lack of energy to get to the lavatory.

4. *Sleeping and Resting*
Noisy breathing and cough disturbs sleep. May be unable to lie down (orthopnoea).

5. *Moving*
Lack of energy affects walking, exercising.

6. *Maintaining Body Temperature*
Dependent on presence/absence of infection.

7. *Keeping Body Clean*
Lack of energy and lack of mental orientation may mean neglect.

8. *Dressing Suitably*
Lack of energy and lack of mental orientation lessens interest.

9. *Avoiding Danger and Injuries*
Lack of energy and lack of mental orientation lessens alertness.

10. *Communicating*
May have difficulty in talking if short of breath, resulting in short sentences.

11. *Worshipping*
Unable to attend public worship due to lack of energy and obtrusive breathing and coughing.

12. *Working*
May be unable to follow normal work, temporarily or permanently.

13. *Participating in Recreation*
Depending on physical activity, change may be necessary.

14. *Learning and Satisfying Curiosity*
Mental activity may be dulled.

## A METHOD TO ASSIST YOU IN ASSESSING MR JONES

In this method we would like you to look at the assessment sheet that follows (*Figure 3.7*) and to complete the top section only at this stage, i.e. consider the conditions always present that affect basic needs. Using the assessment sheet, circle the appropriate features relating to Mr Jones' age, temperament, social setting, capabilities and physiological disturbance. This will help you to complete a personal profile of Mr Jones.

**Figure 3.7** *A patient profile to assist in assessing patients and the development of a problem-solving approach to care*

---

Name _____ Mr Jones _____ No. _____

Address _____

Circle any features that are present in your patient in each of the five columns. Remember that more than one is possible in most of the columns

Section A 1. Starting with the age column, take your selected condition and consider each of the 14 functions requiring assistance and tick in the box(es) those appropriate to your patient's needs, e.g. an elderly patient may require assistance with 2, 3 and 5

Section B 2. Repeat the same procedure with subsequent columns

---

### (A) Conditions always present that affect basic needs

**Physiological disturbances**

| *Age* | *Temperament* | *Social/Cultural* | *Physical/Intellectual Capacity* | |
|---|---|---|---|---|
| Newborn | Emotional state | Member of a family | Normal weight | 1. Fluid and electrolyte imbalance |
| Child | or passing mode: | unit with friends | Over-weight | 2. Oxygen want |
| Adolescent | (a) normal | and status | Under-weight | 3. Shock |
| Adult | (b) euphoric, | A person relatively | Normal mentality | 4. Consciousness |
| Middle aged | hyperactive | alone | Gifted mentality | 5. Local injury/disease |
| Elderly | (c) anxious, fearful, | Maladjusted | Normal sense of: | 6. Metabolism |
| Aged | agitated, | Destitute | hearing | 7. Seeing, hearing, smell and touch |
| | hysterical | Smoker | sight | 8. Communicable conditions |
| | (d) depressed/ | Drinker | equilibrium | 9. Immobilisation: disease/treatment |
| | hypoactive | | touch | |
| | | | Loss of sense of: | |
| | | | hearing | |
| | | | sight | |
| | | | equilibrium | |
| | | | touch | |
| | | | Normal motor power | |
| | | | Loss of motor power | |

### (B)

| Functions requiring assistance | Age | Temperament | Social/Cultural | Physical/Intellectual Capacity | Physiological Disturbance |
|---|---|---|---|---|---|
| 1. Breathing | | | | | |
| 2. Eating or drinking | | | | | |
| 3. Elimination | | | | | |
| 4. Sleep or rest | | | | | |
| 5. Movement | | | | | |
| 6. Maintenance of body temperature | | | | | |
| 7. Keeping body clean | | | | | |
| 8. Dressing suitably | | | | | |
| 9. Avoiding dangers and injury | | | | | |
| 10. Communication | | | | | |
| 11. Worship | | | | | |
| 12. Work | | | | | |
| 13. Participation in recreation | | | | | |
| 14. Learning to satisfy curiosity | | | | | |

Now use this information to decide which of his total needs (physiological, security, achievement and self-fulfilment) may be altered for him as an individual at this time. As a guide refer to the sample profiles in Section 1, Chapter 2, numbers 8, 11 and 15 and decide how Mr Jones is different. Check your ideas with the completed profile, *Figure 3.8*.

**Figure 3.8** *Profile for Mr Jones before admission to hospital*

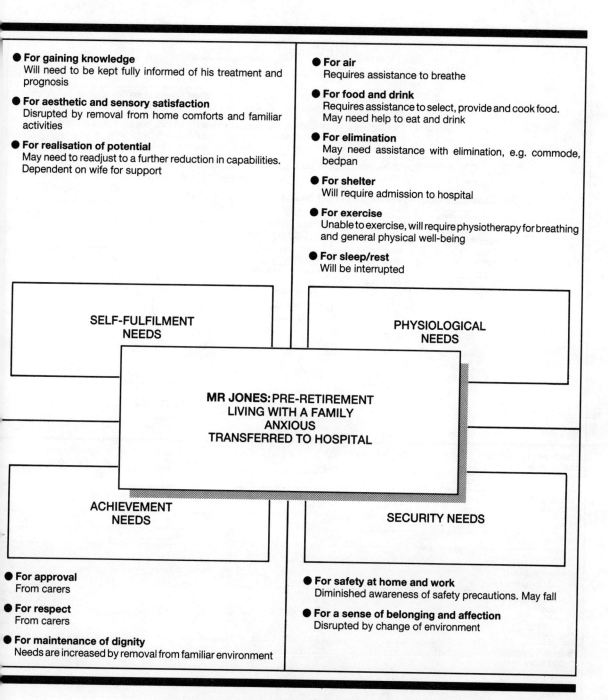

- **For gaining knowledge**
  Will need to be kept fully informed of his treatment and prognosis
- **For aesthetic and sensory satisfaction**
  Disrupted by removal from home comforts and familiar activities
- **For realisation of potential**
  May need to readjust to a further reduction in capabilities. Dependent on wife for support

- **For air**
  Requires assistance to breathe
- **For food and drink**
  Requires assistance to select, provide and cook food. May need help to eat and drink
- **For elimination**
  May need assistance with elimination, e.g. commode, bedpan
- **For shelter**
  Will require admission to hospital
- **For exercise**
  Unable to exercise, will require physiotherapy for breathing and general physical well-being
- **For sleep/rest**
  Will be interrupted

SELF-FULFILMENT NEEDS

PHYSIOLOGICAL NEEDS

MR JONES: PRE-RETIREMENT
LIVING WITH A FAMILY
ANXIOUS
TRANSFERRED TO HOSPITAL

ACHIEVEMENT NEEDS

SECURITY NEEDS

- **For approval**
  From carers
- **For respect**
  From carers
- **For maintenance of dignity**
  Needs are increased by removal from familiar environment

- **For safety at home and work**
  Diminished awareness of safety precautions. May fall
- **For a sense of belonging and affection**
  Disrupted by change of environment

You are now in a position to complete the lower section of the assessment sheet (*Figure 3.7*). Starting with the age column, take your selected feature (previously circled) and consider each of the 14 functions requiring assistance and tick in the box(es) those appropriate to Mr Jones' needs. Repeat the same procedure with the subsequent columns. Check your completed assessment sheet with the sample that follows, *Figure 3.9*.

**Figure 3.9.**   *A patient profile to assist in assessing patients and the development of a problem-solving approach to care*

Name __ Mr Jones _____ No. _____

Address _____

Circle any features that are present in your patient in each of the five columns. Remember that more than one is possible in most of the columns

Section B   1. Starting with the age column, take your selected condition and consider each of the 14 functions requiring assistance and tick in the box(es) those appropriate to your patient's needs, e.g. an elderly patient may require assistance with 2, 3 and 5

Section A   2. Repeat the same procedure with subsequent columns

**(A)   Conditions always present that affect basic needs**

**Physiological disturbances**

| *Age* | *Temperament* | *Social/Cultural* | *Physical/Intellectual Capacity* | |
|---|---|---|---|---|
| Newborn | Emotional state | Member of a family | | 1. Fluid and electrolyte imbalance |
| Child | or passing mode: | unit with friends | Normal weight | 2. Oxygen want |
| Adolescent | (a) normal | and status | Over-weight | 3. Shock |
| Adult | (b) euphoric, | A person relatively | Under-weight | 4. Consciousness |
| Middle aged | hyperactive | alone | Normal mentality | 5. Local injury/ disease |
| Elderly | (c) anxious, fearful, | Maladjusted | Gifted mentality | 6. Metabolism |
| Aged | agitated, | Destitute | Normal sense of: | 7. Seeing, hearing, smell and touch |
| | hysterical | Smoker (Ex.) | hearing | 8. Communicable conditions |
| | (d) depressed/ | Drinker | sight | 9. Immobilisation: disease/treatment |
| | hypoactive | | equilibrium | |
| | | | touch | |
| | | | Loss of sense of: | |
| | | | hearing | |
| | | | sight | |
| | | | equilibrium | |
| | | | touch | |
| | | | Normal motor power | |
| | | | Loss of motor power | |

**(B)**

| **Functions requiring assistance** | *Age* | *Temperament* | *Social/Cultural* | *Physical/Intellectual Capacity* | *Physiological Disturbance* |
|---|---|---|---|---|---|
| 1. Breathing | | ✓ | ✓ | | ✓ |
| 2. Eating or drinking | | | | | ✓ |
| 3. Elimination | | | | | |
| 4. Sleep or rest | | ✓ | | | ✓ |
| 5. Movement | | | | | ✓ |
| 6. Maintenance of body temperature | | | | | ✓ |
| 7. Keeping body clean | | | | | ✓ |
| 8. Dressing suitably | | | | | ✓ |
| 9. Avoiding dangers and injury | | | | | ✓ |
| 10. Communication | | ✓ | | | ✓ |
| 11. Worship | | | | | |
| 12. Work | | | | | ✓ |
| 13. Participation in recreation | | | | | ✓ |
| 14. Learning to satisfy curiosity | | | | | ✓ |

You now know that Mr Jones' temperament, social setting and disease process have a particular effect on his ability to meet his physiological, security, self-fulfilment and achievement needs. From this information you can develop a problem-solving approach to care.

## SELECTING NURSING ACTIONS TO ASSIST A PATIENT WITH DIFFICULTY IN BREATHING

The main problem being discussed in this chapter is *difficulty in breathing*. We would now like you to choose from the list of nursing actions given in *Table 3.2* those appropriate for Mr Jones by putting a tick in either the 'Yes' column if you think the action is appropriate, in the 'No' column if you think the action is inappropriate or dangerous or in the 'Maybe' column if the action is possible. Whatever your decision, give an explanation for each of your choices and when you have completed this compare your decisions and explanations with those given on pages 62–64.

*Table 3.2   Nursing actions to assist a patient with difficulty in breathing*

| Nursing actions | Yes | No | Maybe | Reason for choice |
|---|---|---|---|---|
| **Part 1   Breathing** | | | | |
| 1. Sit the patient upright | | | | |
| 2. Sit supported by pillows | | | | |
| 3. Use backrest to help patient to sit | | | | |
| 4. Sit supported by bed table | | | | |
| 5. Position semi-recumbent | | | | |
| 6. Position lateral | | | | |
| 7. Give oxygen in high concentration | | | | |
| 8. Give oxygen in low concentration | | | | |
| 9. Give oxygen by mask | | | | |
| 10. Oxygen tent | | | | |
| 11. Oxygen by nasal catheter | | | | |
| 12. Give steam inhalation | | | | |
| 13. Give artificial ventilation | | | | |
| 14. Teach breathing exercises | | | | |
| 15. Give postural drainage | | | | |
| 16. Assist expectoration | | | | |

*Table 3.2 Continued*

| Nursing actions | Yes | No | Maybe | Reason for choice |
|---|---|---|---|---|
| **Part 1   Breathing (continued)** | | | | |
| 17. Provide sputum container | | | | |
| 18. Provide tissues | | | | |
| 19. Provide disposal bag | | | | |
| **Part 2   Eating and Drinking** | | | | |
| 1. Provide normal diet | | | | |
| 2. Provide light diet | | | | |
| 3. Provide fluid diet | | | | |
| 4. Assist with eating: cut up food | | | | |
| 5. Assist with actual feeding | | | | |
| 6. Assist with choice of food and drink | | | | |
| 7. Leave menu for patient to complete | | | | |
| 8. Leave jug of drinking water within reach on locker | | | | |
| 9. Remind and offer cool drinks hourly | | | | |
| 10. Offer drink with meals | | | | |
| 11. Give staff and patient guidance on increasing fluid intake | | | | |
| 12. Give guidance to staff and patient on decreasing fluid intake | | | | |
| 13. Give mouthwashes | | | | |
| 14. Perform oral toilet | | | | |
| 15. Encourage patient to brush own teeth | | | | |
| **Part 3   Eliminating** | | | | |
| 1. Allow patient to go to toilet as required | | | | |
| 2. Provide commode during day | | | | |
| 3. Provide commode at night | | | | |
| 4. Give bedpans/urinals | | | | |

*Table 3.2 Continued*

| Nursing actions | Yes | No | Maybe | Reason for choice |
|---|---|---|---|---|
| **Part 4   Sleeping and Resting** | | | | |
| 1. Keep patient awake during the day to ensure a night's sleep | | | | |
| 2. Offer warm drink at night | | | | |
| 3. Ensure adequate ventilation in the ward | | | | |
| 4. Position patient's bed in main ward | | | | |
| 5. Position bed in cubicle (side ward) | | | | |
| 6. Position bed near nurses' station | | | | |
| **Part 5   Moving** | | | | |
| 1. Keep patient at complete rest | | | | |
| 2. Encourage exercise | | | | |
| 3. Sit in easy chair | | | | |
| 4. Assist in repositioning in bed | | | | |
| 5. Provide sheepskin | | | | |
| 6. Provide ripple bed | | | | |
| 7. Provide hoist | | | | |
| **Part 6   Maintaining Body Temperature** | | | | |
| 1. Provide plenty of blankets | | | | |
| 2. Provide light bedclothes | | | | |
| 3. Provide bed cradle | | | | |
| 4. Open nearby windows | | | | |
| 5. Turn radiators on full | | | | |
| 6. Use electric fan | | | | |
| **Part 7   Keeping Body Clean** | | | | |
| 1. Give daily bed bath | | | | |
| 2. Assist patient to wash in bed | | | | |
| 3. Assist patient to wash in bathroom | | | | |

*Table 3.2 Continued*

| Nursing actions | Yes | No | Maybe | Reason for choice |
|---|---|---|---|---|
| **Part 7   Keeping Body Clean (continued)** | | | | |
| 4. Encourage patient to bath himself | | | | |
| 5. Assist patient to shave, and brush hair | | | | |
| 6. Leave shaving until patient feels better | | | | |
| **Part 8   Dressing Suitably** | | | | |
| 1. Provide hospital pyjamas | | | | |
| 2. Provide hospital gown | | | | |
| 3. Encourage use of own pyjamas | | | | |
| 4. Encourage use of dressing gown and slippers | | | | |
| **Part 9   Avoiding Dangers and Injury** | | | | |
| 1. Position locker within reach | | | | |
| 2. Position locker out of reach to prevent accidents | | | | |
| 3. Fix cotside during day | | | | |
| 4. Fix cotside during night | | | | |
| 5. Anticipate patient's requirements | | | | |
| 6. Encourage patient to ask for what he wants | | | | |
| 7. Administer antibiotics, bronchodilators and expectorant as prescribed | | | | |
| 8. Ensure all are aware of the precautions to be taken during administration of oxygen | | | | |
| **Part 10   Communicating** | | | | |
| 1. Provide communication (call) bell | | | | |
| 2. Provide notepad and pencil | | | | |
| 3. Provide distress flares | | | | |
| 4. Allocate a nurse to the patient | | | | |
| 5. Encourage wife to assist with care | | | | |
| 6. Offer relatives accommodation | | | | |
| 7. Encourage free visiting | | | | |

*Table 3.2 Continued*

| Nursing actions | Yes | No | Maybe | Reason for choice |
|---|---|---|---|---|
| **Part 10   Communicating (continued)** | | | | |
| 8. Limit visiting | | | | |
| 9. Exchange tel. nos. for contact during day and/or night | | | | |
| 10. Explain progress and treatment to patient only | | | | |
| 11. Explain progress and treatment to patient's wife | | | | |
| 12. Explain progress and treatment to wife only | | | | |
| 13. Give opportunity for exchange of information between patient/staff/relatives | | | | |
| 14. Provide Health Education when patient's condition allows | | | | |
| **Part 11   Worshipping** | | | | |
| 1. Inform hospital chaplain | | | | |
| 2. Inform patient's own chaplain of patient's admission | | | | |
| 3. Ignore spiritual needs until patient is feeling better | | | | |
| **Part 12   Working** | | | | |
| 1. Inform patient's employers | | | | |
| 2. Contact medical social worker | | | | |
| 3. Contact rehabilitation officer | | | | |
| 4. Wait to inform the above until prognosis is clearer | | | | |
| **Parts 13 and 14   Participating in Recreation and Learning to Satisfy Curiosity** | | | | |
| 1. Assist patient in getting daily paper | | | | |
| 2. Read patient's personal mail to him | | | | |
| 3. Provide formal occupational therapy | | | | |
| 4. Keep patient fully informed of his condition and progress | | | | |

## EXPLANATION FOR CHOICE OF NURSING ACTIONS

### Part 1   Breathing

We hope you have ticked the Yes column for numbers 1, 2, 3, 8, 14, 16, 17, 18, 19. These actions would help Mr Jones to breathe more easily. By sitting him upright he could more fully expand the thoracic cavity. Oxygen therapy in low concentration is essential to improve arterial oxygen level without depressing the reflex stimulus to respiration which is caused by reduced blood oxygen levels. By teaching breathing exercises Mr Jones can improve his respiratory function. As he is ill he may need help to cough up sputum, therefore sputum container, tissues and disposal bag must be provided for observation and safe disposal.

You may have ticked the Maybe column for number 4. If Mr Jones is very weak he may find relief from leaning forward resting on a bed table which can increase chest expansion by lifting the rib cage. For number 5 it may be possible to position Mr Jones semi-recumbant for periods of rest. Numbers 9 and 11: oxygen may appropriately be given by either method and may be determined by whichever method is tolerated by Mr Jones. Number 15, postural drainage, can help to clear the bases of the lungs of excessive sputum which might otherwise be difficult to expectorate.

You should have ticked the No column for numbers 6, 7, 10, 12 and 13. The lateral position prevents expansion of both lungs and should only be used as part of postural drainage. A high concentration of oxygen should never be used for a patient with chronic bronchitis as it reduces the respiratory drive of reduced arterial oxygen level. The use of an oxygen tent would not be appropriate for an adult. Steam inhalations have a debatable value for bronchitis and are potentially dangerous. Artificial ventilation is not appropriate, even in severe respiratory difficulties from bronchitis as it has the risk of being a long-term need and does not necessarily assist in rehabilitation.

### Part 2   Eating and Drinking

We hope you have ticked the Yes column for numbers 2, 6, 9, 11 and 13. Because of Mr Jones' breathing difficulties he will be able to manage a light diet only and should therefore be assisted with his food and drink. He should be offered cool drinks frequently to combat loss of fluid due to pyrexia, rapid respiration and production of sputum. Overall fluid intake will be increased and mouthwashes are necessary since receiving oxygen can dry the mucous membranes.

You may have ticked the Maybe column for numbers 3, 4, 8, 10, 14, 15. If Mr Jones is very weak he may need his food cut up or he may only manage a fluid diet. He may not be able to lift and pour from a jug of drinking water left on the locker and if offered drinks with meals this may further depress his appetite. If he is unable to brush his own teeth he may need oral toilet. You should have ticked numbers 1, 5, 7 and 12 in the No column. Mr Jones will not be able to tolerate a normal diet though he should be able to feed himself. There would be no point in leaving the menu for him to complete as he would not be particularly interested or able. Fluid intake should be sufficient to replace fluid loss and to maintain hydration.

### Part 3    Eliminating

We hope you have ticked the Yes column for number 4 as Mr Jones would be too weak to tolerate alternatives. It may be possible for him to use the commode with help during the day.

### Part 4    Sleeping and Resting

We hope you have ticked the Yes column for numbers 2, 3, 4 and 6. Offering a warm drink at night could assist Mr Jones to relax and sleep and gives extra nutrition and fluids. Adequate ventilation in the ward keeps the air fresh and pleasant. Mr Jones can be more easily observed if he is in the main ward near the Nurses' Station. The No column should have been ticked for numbers 1 and 5. Keeping the patient awake during the day reduces the opportunities for rest and recovery. Intensive therapy will be carried out throughout the 24 hours so Mr Jones should be allowed to sleep and rest when he can.

### Part 5    Moving

We hope you have ticked the Yes column for numbers 4 and 5. During his acute illness Mr Jones will be confined to bed and will require assistance in moving to promote comfort and reduce risk of pressure sores. Providing a sheepskin will reduce pressure and friction to Mr Jones' sacral area. In the Maybe column you should have ticked 2, 3, 6 and 7. Even if confined to bed Mr Jones should be helped to exercise his limbs to aid venous return and prevent deep vein thrombosis. Depending on his condition he may find breathing easier sitting in a chair providing he is kept warm. If he is very ill and weak he may find it more comfortable on a ripplebed and for a hoist to be used. The No column should have been ticked for number 1 as complete rest could increase the risks of hypostatic pneumonia, venous stasis, loss of muscle tone and mental apathy.

### Part 6    Maintaining Body Temperature

We hope you have ticked in the Yes column for number 2 since this action with numbers 3 and 6 in the Maybe column would assist in keeping Mr Jones comfortable and prevent overheating. You should have ticked numbers 1, 4 and 5 in the No column. Too many blankets could restrict chest and leg movements while opening the windows creates draughts and turning the radiators on full could overheat Mr Jones.

### Part 7    Keeping Body Clean

We hope you have ticked in the Yes column numbers 2 and 5 as these would assist in maintaining Mr Jones' dignity, independence and personal hygiene. It could be possible that Mr Jones would be weak enough to require a daily bed bath. For the No column you should have ticked numbers 3, 4 and 6. He is unlikely to be well enough to go to the bathroom and so will need assistance and should be helped to shave regularly.

### Part 8    Dressing Suitably

We hope you have ticked in the Yes column for number 3 to assist in maintaining Mr Jones' identity while in hospital. Hospital pyjamas or a gown may be used for Mr Jones while he is febrile and weak. Dressing gown and slippers may be necessary, Yes for number 4, if he is able to sit out in a chair or use a commode.

### Part 9    Avoiding Danger or Injury

We hope you have ticked in the Yes column numbers 1, 5, 6, 7 and 8. By positioning the locker within reach and encouraging Mr Jones to ask for what he wants you can maintain his sense of independence while encouraging a safe environment. By administering the medicines as prescribed you are assuring the appropriate treatment is being received and you must ensure safety by following the procedure for protection of patients, staff and visitors during oxygen administration. You should have ticked number 2 in the No column as this will reduce Mr Jones' independence and it may be dangerous for him to try to reach the locker. In the Maybe column numbers 3 and 4 may be appropriate to prevent Mr Jones falling if he is mentally disorientated and/or weak.

### Part 10    Communicating

We hope you have ticked in the Yes column numbers 1, 4, 5, 7, 9, 11, 13 and 14. Provision of 1 and 4 assists in promoting Mr Jones' security. One nurse allocated to Mr Jones' care helps in continuity and monitoring of care. Numbers 5 and 7 maintains family contact and helps to develop Mrs Jones knowledge and skills. Number 9 is essential so that a communication link can be established and used in an emergency. Numbers 10 and 13 reduce fears and anxieties and assist in the gaining of cooperation. Number 14 helps in the understanding of Mr Jones' condition and can assist in establishing a reasonable quality of life. In the Maybe column you should have ticked numbers 2, 6 and 8. Number 2 may help if Mr Jones is too breathless to talk without distress. Numbers 6 and 8 may be appropriate if Mr Jones' condition is poor. The only items in the No column are numbers 10 and 12; exclusion of one or other can lead to misunderstanding between Mr and Mrs Jones. Number 3 is for use in distress at sea *only*.

### Part 11    Worshipping

Numbers 1 and 2 could have been ticked in the Maybe column depending upon the patient's wishes. If acknowledged by the patient spiritual needs should be met promptly.

### Part 12    Working

We hope you have ticked the Yes column for number 2 only as, initially, the medical social worker will discuss with Mr Jones and his wife the course of action required for employment and rehabilitation.

### Parts 13 and 14    Participating in Recreation and Learning to Satisfy Curiosity

You should have ticked number 4 in the Yes column. Numbers 1 and 2 may be appropriate in assisting in keeping in contact with outside affairs. Formal occupational therapy is not appropriate at this stage though it may be used eventually to assess for rehabilitation.

### Discussion and Questioning

We hope that you have grasped that some nursing actions are wholly dependent on the individual characteristics of the patient and the particular time and place so they cannot be applied routinely to all patients. Therefore care plans need to be sensitive to the individual patient's needs. If you disagree strongly with some of the answers we have suggested perhaps you would like to discuss them further with your colleagues and Tutor. This will help you to develop a questioning approach to nursing care with a view to checking on standards of care and nursing practice.

This list you have just considered is in no particular order of importance. For successful planning of the care that Mr Jones requires you will need to identify priorities, that is, which aspects of care require prompt attention and which aspects may be safely left for later consideration.

## CHOOSING PRIORITIES IN NURSING ACTIONS

*Table 3.3* is the list of V. Henderson's Components of basic nursing care used in Parts 1–14.

*Table 3.3   Priorities in nursing actions*

| Part | Insert your choice of priority: numbers 1–14 |
|---|---|
| 1.  Breathing | |
| 2.  Eating and drinking | |
| 3.  Eliminating | |
| 4.  Sleeping and resting | |
| 5.  Moving | |
| 6.  Maintaining body temperature | |
| 7.  Keeping body clean | |
| 8.  Dressing suitably | |
| 9.  Avoiding dangers and injury | |
| 10.  Communicating | |
| 11.  Worshipping | |
| 12.  Working | |
| 13.  Participation in recreation | |
| 14.  Learning to satisfy curiosity | |

We would now like you to number each of the components you would consider in order of priority, bearing in mind the aspects that are potentially life threatening, e.g. difficulty in breathing, those that help to maintain the patient's and relatives' peace of mind and those that can be left until a more convenient time, e.g. keeping the body clean and recreation. You can now check your decisions with the plan shown in *Table 3.5*.

As you can see, Part 1 Breathing is considered to be first priority with Part 10 Communicating, Part 11 Worshipping and Part 14 Satisfying Curiosity as joint second priorities. Check your subsequent sequence with *Table 3.5*. Don't be surprised if you find some differences of opinion, as long as you can justify your decision without jeopardising your patient's safety and well-being.

Table 3.4    *Necessary actions in planning and providing nursing care*

|  | Please refer to headings of columns on Plan of Care |
|---|---|
| ● Decide on appropriate care | Yes |
| ● Decide on potential care | Maybe |
| ● Decide on what to do first, second and third, etc. | Priority choice |
| ● Decide which observations or measurements are needed to adequately monitor patient's progress | Measurements |
| ● Select realistic outcomes | Short-term goals |
| ● Decide when to review results of Nursing Actions | Review period |
| ● Give opportunity for stating results of evaluation and possible alteration of short-term goals and review period | Evaluation criteria |

## IDENTIFICATION OF CRITERIA FOR PROGRESS

Now read carefully the plan shown in *Table 3.5* identifying criteria for progress.

*Table 3.5 Plan of care for progress*

| Nursing actions to assist a patient with difficulty in breathing. | Yes | Maybe | Priority Choice | Measurements | Short-term goals | Review period | Evaluation criteria Have short-term goals been met? |
|---|---|---|---|---|---|---|---|
| **Part 1 Breathing** | | | | Note: | | | |
| 1. Sit the patient upright | ✓ | | | (a) Rate, depth and difficulty in breathing | (a) Reduction in respiratory rate | | (a) Reduction of respiration rate and increase in depth. |
| 2. Sit supported by pillows | ✓ | | | (b) Skin and mucous membranes for cyanosis | (b) No presence of cyanosis | Hourly | (b) Colour grey |
| 3. Sit supported by backrest | ✓ | | | (c) Character of cough | (c) Expectoration easier | | (c) Cough still present |
| 4. Sit supported by bed table | | ✓ | | (d) Texture, colour, amount of sputum | (d) Expectoration easier | 4-hourly | (d) Sputum less tenacious. Volume increased |
| 5. Position semi-recumbant | | ✓ | | (e) Rate and concentration oxygen therapy. | (e) Required less frequently | | (e) Requires intermittent oxygen therapy |
| 8. O$_2$ therapy in low concentration | ✓ | | | Assist and record: | | Hourly | |
| 9. O$_2$ by mask | | ✓ | | (f) Assist medical staff in obtaining sputum specimen for pathological investigation | (f) To obtain second specimen if required | | (f) Sputum specimen collected to await result |
| 11. O$_2$ by nasal catheter | | ✓ | | | | | |
| 14. Teach breathing exercises | ✓ | | | | | | |
| 15. Give postural drainage | | ✓ | | (g) Record results peak flow, forced expiratory volume | (g) Results should be maintained or improved | | (g) Peak flow. Slight improvement only |
| 16. Assist expectoration | ✓ | | | (h) Assist medical staff in obtaining blood samples for measurement of haemoglobin, white cell count, PCO$_2$ and PO$_2$ | (h) Obtain 2nd specimen if required, show improvement or maintenance | Within first 24 hours | (h) Slight improvement only |
| 17. Provide sputum container | ✓ | | | | | | |
| 18. Provide tissues | ✓ | | | | | | |
| 19. Provide disposal bag | ✓ | | | Chest X-ray | Results may show lung fields clearer | | Slight improvement only |

(Priority Choice column spans items 1–19 bracketed as **FIRST**)

*Table 3.5 Continued*

| Nursing actions to assist a patient with difficulty in breathing. | Yes | Maybe | Priority Choice | Measurements | Short-term goals | Review period | Evaluation criteria Have short-term goals been met? |
|---|---|---|---|---|---|---|---|
| **Part 10 Communicating**<br><br>1. Provide communication (call) bell | ✓ | | SECOND | Note level of anxiety/frustration from patient and relatives | Both Mr and Mrs Jones confident in the care being given | Within first 24 hours | Mr and Mrs Jones to be informed of current results<br><br>Satisfactory visiting arrangements as Mrs Jones wishes to be contacted day or night |
| 2. Provide notepad and pencil | | ✓ | | | | | |
| 4. Allocate a nurse to the patient | ✓ | | | | | | |
| 5. Encourage wife to assist with care | ✓ | | | | | | |
| 6. Offer relatives accommodation | | ✓ | | | | | |
| 7. Encourage free visiting | ✓ | | | | | | |
| 8. Limit visiting | | ✓ | | | | | |
| 9. Exchange tel. nos for contact day and night | ✓ | | | | | | |
| 10 and 11. Explain progress and treatment to patient and wife | ✓ | | | | | | |
| 13. Give opportunity for exchange of information between patient/staff/relatives | ✓ | | | | | | |
| 14. Provide health education when patient's condition allows | ✓ | | | | | | |
| **Part 11  Worship**<br><br>1. Inform hospital chaplain | | ✓ | SECOND | Note Mr Jones' desire for spiritual help | Satisfaction of spiritual needs if necessary | Within first 24 hours | Link established with hospital chaplain |
| 2. Inform patient's own chaplain | | ✓ | | | | | |

*Table 3.5 Continued*

| Nursing actions to assist a patient with difficulty in breathing. | Yes | Maybe | Priority Choice | Measurements | Short-term goals | Review period | Evaluation criteria Have short-term goals been met? |
|---|---|---|---|---|---|---|---|
| **Part 13 Participating in Recreation and Part 14 Learning to Satisfy Curiosity** | | | SECOND | Note Mr Jones' orientation to time and place | Mr Jones orientated to present setting | Within first 24 hours | Not yet interested in daily events. Wife dealing with personal mail |
| 1. Assist patient in getting daily paper | | ✓ | | | | | |
| 2. Read patient's mail to him | | ✓ | | | | | |
| 4. Keep patient fully informed of his condition and progress | ✓ | | | | | | |
| **Part 4 Sleeping and Resting** | | | THIRD | Note sleep pattern and periods of wakefulness, rest and sleep | Allow short periods of sleep and comfort | Within first 24 hours | Mr Jones sleeps for short periods only |
| 2. Offer warm drink at night | ✓ | | | | | | |
| 3. Ensure adequate ventilation in ward | ✓ | | | | | | |
| 4. Position patient's bed in main ward | ✓ | | | | | | |
| 6. Position patient's bed near nurses' station | ✓ | | | | | | |
| **Part 6 Maintaining Body Temperature** | | | FOURTH | Note the body temperature, presence of sweat | To reduce body temperature to within normal limits | Every 4 hours in the first 24 hours | Temperature still elevated. Sweating reduced |
| 2. Provide light bedclothes | ✓ | | | | | | |
| 3. Provide bed cradle | | ✓ | | | | | |
| 6. Use electric fan | | ✓ | | | | | |

*Table 3.5 Continued*

| Nursing actions to assist a patient with difficulty in breathing. | Yes | Maybe | Priority Choice | Measurements | Short-term goals | Review period | Evaluation Criteria Have short-term goals been met? |
|---|---|---|---|---|---|---|---|
| **Part 9   Avoiding Danger and Injury** | | | FIFTH | (a) Note the potential hazards of obstacles at bedside | (a) Protection from accident or incident | Hourly while in dependant state | (a) No accident or incident |
| 1. Position locker within reach | ✓ | | | | | | |
| 3. Fix cotsides during day | | ✓ | | (b) Note the unwanted effects of *antibiotics*, i.e. presence of rashes, nausea, fungal infections, constipation, diarrhoea | (b) Early detection of unwanted effects of medicines | Hourly during first 24 hours | (b) No unwanted effects of medicines |
| 4. Fix cotsides during night | | ✓ | | | | | |
| 5. Anticipate patient's requirements | ✓ | | | | | | |
| 6. Encourage patient to ask for what he needs | ✓ | | | *Bronchial dilators*, i.e. drop in blood pressure | | | |
| 7. Administer antibiotics, bronchodilators and expectorant as prescribed | ✓ | | | *Oxygen therapy* for confusion, anoxia, respiratory arrest | | | |
| 8. Ensure all are aware of the precautions to be taken during administration of oxygen | ✓ | | | | | | |
| **Part 5   Moving** | | | SIXTH | Note early signs and symptoms of complications of immobility/inspect pressure sites for redness, abrasions. Check range of movement of all joints | To avoid complications of immobility | Every 2 hours within the first 24 hours | Pressure areas are intact, no evidence of calf tenderness, capable of exercising in bed |
| 2. Encourage exercise | | ✓ | | | | | |
| 3. Sit in easy chair | | ✓ | | | | | |
| 4. Assist in repositioning in bed | ✓ | | | | | | |
| 5. Provide sheepskin | ✓ | | | | | | |
| 6. Provide ripple bed | | ✓ | | | | | |
| 7. Provide hoist | | ✓ | | | | | |

*Table 3.5 Continued*

| Nursing actions to assist a patient with difficulty in breathing. | Yes | Maybe | Priority Choice | Measurements | Short-term goals | Review period | Evaluation criteria Have short-term goals been met? |
|---|---|---|---|---|---|---|---|
| **Part 2  Eating and Drinking** | | | | (a) Record fluid intake, note nutritional intake, state of hunger and thirst | Patient should have drunk total 3 litres fluid and consumed minimum 1500 calories within 24 hours | Every 8 hours within 1st 24 hours | Patient managed to consume 3 litres of fluids but still having difficulty eating. Calorie intake insufficient |
| 2. Provide light diet | ✓ | | | | | | |
| 3. Provide fluid diet | | ✓ | | | | | |
| 4. Assist with eating: cut up food | | ✓ | | | | | |
| 6. Assist with choice | ✓ | | | | | | |
| 8. Leave jug of drinking water | | ✓ | SEVENTH | (b) check state of oral hygiene | A moist healthy mouth | Every 4 hours in the first 24 hours | Lips cracked and tongue dry and coated |
| 9. Remind and offer cool drinks hourly | ✓ | | | | | | |
| 10. Offer drink with meals | | ✓ | | | | | |
| 11. Give staff and patient guidance whether fluid intake should be increased | ✓ | | | | | | |
| 13. Give mouth washes | ✓ | | | | | | |
| 14. Perform oral toilet | | ✓ | | | | | |
| 15. Encourage patient to brush own teeth | | ✓ | | | | | |
| **Part 3  Eliminating** | | | EIGHTH | (a) Measure and record fluid output. Estimate insensible loss from sweating and respiration | 24-hourly urine output of 1½ litres | 8-hourly within first 24 hours | 24-hour total 1 litre |
| 2. Provide commode during day | | ✓ | | | | | |
| 4. Give bedpans/ urinals | ✓ | | | (b) Note consistency and frequency of bowel action | Maintain usual bowel action | 24-hourly | No bowel action since admission |
| **Part 7  Keeping the Body Clean** | | | NINTH | (a) Note the patient's ability to care for his own hygiene | Maintain cleanliness during period of dependance | 24-hourly | Still requires help with majority of washing in bed |
| 1. Give daily bed bath | | ✓ | | | | 24-hourly | |
| 2. Assist patient washing in bed | ✓ | | | (b) Note state of skin, hair and nails | Maintain good condition of skin, hair and nails | | State of skin satisfactory. Hair requires washing |
| 5. Assist patient to shave, and brush hair | ✓ | | | | | | |

*Table 3.5 Continued*

| Nursing actions to assist a patient with difficulty in breathing. | Yes | Maybe | Priority Choice | Measurements | Short-term goals | Review period | Evaluation criteria Have short-term goals been met? |
|---|---|---|---|---|---|---|---|
| **Part 8   Dressing Suitably**<br><br>1. Provide hospital pyjamas<br><br>2. Provide hospital gown<br><br>3. Encourage use of own pyjamas<br><br>4. Encourage use of dressing gown and slippers | | ✓<br><br>✓<br><br><br>✓ (3)<br><br>✓ | } TENTH | Check patient is dressed appropriately to his body temperature, environment and level of activity | Ensure patient not overheated or cooled by clothing | Every 4 hours within first 24 hours | Still needs frequent change of clothing |
| **Part 12   Participating in Work**<br><br>2. Contact medical social worker | | | } ELEVENTH | Note any social or work-related problems that require assistance | Mr and Mrs Jones have no immediate worries about the effects of Mr Jones' illness | 2 days after admission | Medical social worker in contact with Mr and Mrs Jones |

*Note: in Part 8 the ✓ for "3. Encourage use of own pyjamas" appears in the Yes column; Part 12 "2. Contact medical social worker" ✓ appears in the Yes column.*

### Using Evaluation Criteria for Resetting Short-term Goals

Using a plan such as *Table 3.5* with evaluation criteria illustrates that Nursing Care Planning is a dynamic process. By using appropriate review periods of patient's progress it is easy to identify which aspects of the patient's progress have improved and therefore need less nursing assistance, those aspects which remain the same and therefore need continuation of nursing assistance and those which have deteriorated and need different nursing assistance. The Nursing Care Plan needs to be altered as the patient's progress changes with identification of new short-term goals.

### IDENTIFICATION OF LONG-TERM GOALS

Long-term goals should be identified to enable Mr Jones to function at home with some assistance from others. As he has a long-term illness it would be unrealistic to expect him to regain total independence. If you remember the individual profiles in Section 1 you should be able to prepare a profile of Mr Jones which will indicate his expected level of independence as a long-term goal. You may like to compare this long-term goal profile (*Figure 3.10*) with the one you prepared on admission to hospital as a tool for identifying his needs when he was ill (*Figure 3.8*).

**Figure 3.10**    *Long-Term Goal Profile for Mr Jones*

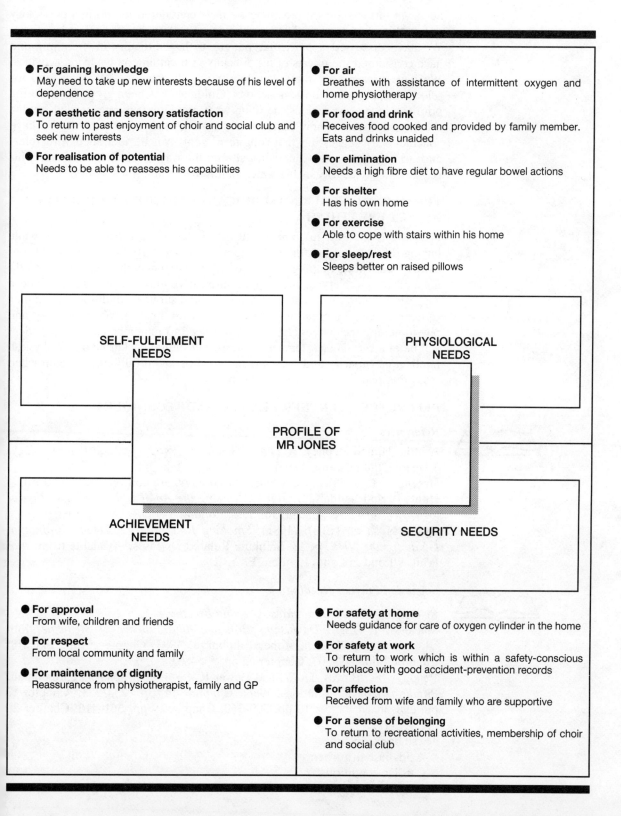

● **For gaining knowledge**
May need to take up new interests because of his level of dependence

● **For aesthetic and sensory satisfaction**
To return to past enjoyment of choir and social club and seek new interests

● **For realisation of potential**
Needs to be able to reassess his capabilities

● **For air**
Breathes with assistance of intermittent oxygen and home physiotherapy

● **For food and drink**
Receives food cooked and provided by family member. Eats and drinks unaided

● **For elimination**
Needs a high fibre diet to have regular bowel actions

● **For shelter**
Has his own home

● **For exercise**
Able to cope with stairs within his home

● **For sleep/rest**
Sleeps better on raised pillows

SELF-FULFILMENT NEEDS

PHYSIOLOGICAL NEEDS

PROFILE OF MR JONES

ACHIEVEMENT NEEDS

SECURITY NEEDS

● **For approval**
From wife, children and friends

● **For respect**
From local community and family

● **For maintenance of dignity**
Reassurance from physiotherapist, family and GP

● **For safety at home**
Needs guidance for care of oxygen cylinder in the home

● **For safety at work**
To return to work which is within a safety-conscious workplace with good accident-prevention records

● **For affection**
Received from wife and family who are supportive

● **For a sense of belonging**
To return to recreational activities, membership of choir and social club

## SUMMARY NOTES

So far in this chapter on breathing we have considered the normal physiology of breathing and the social and psychological factors that can affect breathing. We have discussed a particular patient with a difficulty in breathing and have considered the effects of his difficulty in breathing on his living activities. We have presented a method to assist you in assessing Mr Jones and for selecting appropriate nursing actions. Guidance has been given for choosing priorities in nursing actions, deciding what measurements are needed, setting short-term goals, review periods, and stating evaluation criteria. We have concluded by suggesting that long-term goals can be identified with reference to how this recent illness has altered the way in which he can satisfy his physiological, security, achievement and self-fulfilment needs.

## FURTHER MEDICAL AND SURGICAL CONDITIONS WHICH MAY AFFECT BREATHING

We have looked at, in some detail, Mr Jones' need for nursing care while having difficulty in breathing during an acute exacerbation of chronic bronchitis. You will be helping to care for other patients with difficulty in breathing due to a variety of medical or surgical conditions. We now include a suggested reading list of common medical and surgical conditions which may cause difficulty in breathing, together with outlines of pharmacology and physiotherapy techniques. However, you need to remember that each patient will be of a certain age, temperament, social/cultural background and physical/ intellectual capacity and these factors must be taken fully into account when assessing, planning and reviewing care.

## REFERENCES, FURTHER READING AND TECHNIQUES

### References

Ashton, H. and Stepney, R. (1982). *Smoking—Psychology and Pharmacology*. Tavistock Publications, London.

Green, J. H. (1978). *Basic Clinical Physiology*, 3rd edition. OUP, Oxford.

Hunt, P. and Sendell, B. (1983). *Nursing the Adult with a Specific Physiological Disturbance*. Macmillan Press, London.

Olsen, N. *et al.* (Eds). (1981). *Smoking Prevention: A Health Promotion Guide for the NHS*, p. 18: Smoking Related Diseases. Available from: Ace Print, 9 London Lane, London, E8 5PR.

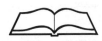

### Suggested Further Reading

*Related to Medical Conditions Affecting Breathing*

Macleod, J. (Ed.). *Davidson's Principles and Practice of Medicine*, 13th edition. Churchill Livingstone, Edinburgh, 1983: Chapter 6 pp. 145–218; Chapter 7 pp. 219–307; Chapter 12 pp. 535–603.

Read, A .E., Barritt, D. W. and Hewer R. L. *Modern Medicine*, 3rd edition. Pitman Medical, London, 1984: Chapter 14 pp. 238–253; Chapter 17 pp. 298–308; Chapter 18 pp. 309–360; Chapter 19 pp. 361–416; Chapter 20 pp. 417–471.

These books include:
● Acid–base disturbance
● Cardiac conditions
● Respiratory conditions

● Disorders of blood and oxygen-carrying capacity
● Poisoning and respiratory depression

*Related to Surgical Conditions Affecting Breathing*
Ellis, H. and Wastell, C. *General Surgery for Nurses.* Blackwell Scientific, Oxford, 1980: Chapter 6 pp. 70–86; Chapter 7 pp. 87–99; Chapter 20 pp. 471–481.
Henderson, M. A. *Essential Surgery for Nurses.* Churchill Livingstone, Oxford, 1980; Chapter 16 pp. 62–66; Chapter 18 pp. 77–86.
Horton, R. *General Surgery and the Nurse.* Hodder and Stoughton, 1983: Chapter 22 pp. 215–218; Chapter 23 pp. 233–234.
These books include:
● Injuries to ribs and lungs
● Lung infections
● Neoplasma of lung and bronchi
● Principles of cardiac surgery
● Surgical conditions of the heart and great vessels
● Pneumothorax
● Haemothorax
● Injuries and tumour of the larynx
● Management of tracheostomy

**Pharmacology and Physiotherapy Techniques Related to Care of Patients with Difficulty in Breathing**
*Medicines*
You may wish to familiarise yourself with the medicines commonly used for patients with difficulty in breathing  e.g.
● Bronchial dilators
● Expectorants
● Antibiotics
See Boyd, G. (1984). *Drugs and the Respiratory System.* Nursing Medical Education, page 805.

*Physiotherapy to Chest*
See Thompson, M. (1982). *Physiotherapy—Essentials of Chest Care.* Nursing Medical Education, page 796.

**Suggested Nursing Procedures / Guidelines for Nursing Practice**
You may wish to familiarise yourself with your local policies and procedures which may be applicable to a patient requiring assistance with difficulty in breathing. Here is a suggested list:
● Chest aspiration
● Insertion of chest drain
● Removal of chest drain
● Oxygen therapy
● Suggested technique of arousal for respiratory failure
● Use of nebulisers
● Tracheostomy and tracheal suction
● Intermittent positive pressure ventilation

*Investigations*
See Twohig, R. G. (1984). *Respiratory Function Tests*, Medical Education (International) Ltd, page 807.

# Chapter 4
# Eating and Drinking

## NORMAL PHYSIOLOGY

Before proceeding we suggest you revise your knowledge of ingestion, digestion, absorption and assimilation by using the following references or any other suitable textbook.

- Hunt and Sendell (1987). *Nursing the Adult with a Specific Physiological Disturbance*, 2nd edn.
- Green (1978). *Basic Clinical Physiology*, pages 74–86 and 92–106.

## SOCIOLOGICAL FACTORS AFFECTING EATING AND DRINKING

Eating and drinking is affected by the availability of abundant nutritious food, the provision of clean and sufficient water and the health and knowledge of the individual. Societies vary as to how they are able to provide sufficient nutritious food and clean water. Legislation has been passed to ensure a safe food supply: the Food and Drugs Act 1955 for England and Wales with similar legislation for Scotland and Northern Ireland; the Bread and Flour Regulations 1963; and the Margarine Regulation in 1967. Sometimes society's provision of suitable food and water can be disrupted by catastrophies and natural disasters such as war, flood, drought, earthquakes or fire, e.g. famine in Ethiopia, burst water main causing water shortage in Yorkshire.

The individual can become more vulnerable in his ability to eat, drink, select and prepare his own food if he lacks the knowledge to select a suitable diet and if he is subjected to restrictive and/or religious practices. The vulnerability is increased if he is unable to select, prepare his own food, and eat and drink due to illness or disability.

It needs to be remembered that the offering and sharing of food and drink is a social activity and is used to celebrate anniversaries, meetings, departures and friendships. Some members of society may be more susceptible to eating and drinking difficulties due to their age, their ability to provide and select adequate food and their state of health enabling them to eat and drink normally. Others may experience difficulty due to the lack of clean water and nutritious food.

If we measure the vulnerability of the individual on the scale 1 to 10 with 1 being the least vulnerable (the more able) and 10 being the most vulnerable (less able) and we measure the availability of clean water and nutritious food on a scale 1 to 10 with 1 being the most available and 10 being the least, we can use the following chart (Figure 4.1) to illustrate how the availability of clean water and nutritious food and the vulnerability of the individual can affect eating and drinking.

**Figure 4.1**  *Chart to illustrate the interrelationships of clean water and nutritious food and the vulnerability of the individual*

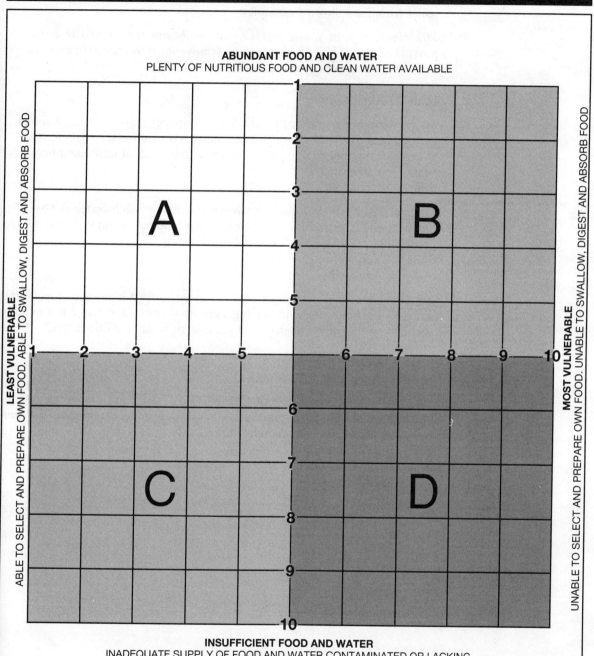

### Interrelationship of Availability of Sufficient Clean Water and Nutritious Food with the Vulnerability of the Individual

We would like you to use the chart as a graph by inserting an 'X' using the two scales from the following examples:

*Mrs Harris* is a fit young mother, with sufficient money and resources to provide a balanced diet for her healthy family. She is interested in cooking and making the best use of what is available.

Scale 1    Vulnerability
Scale 2    Availability

*Mr Edwards* is a generally fit and active newspaper reporter, who, while on a consignment overseas, although aware of what is required for a balanced diet is able to obtain only small amounts of unfamiliar foods at infrequent intervals.

Scale 2    Vulnerability
Scale 8    Availability

*Mrs Davis* is an elderly widow who lives alone, living mainly on tea and biscuits. She is fit and able to shop and cook her own food but doesn't understand the importance of certain foods in a balanced diet.

Scale 8    Vulnerability
Scale 3    Availability

*Mr Thomas* is an elderly man who is unable to feed himself and has some difficulty in swallowing since having a cerebrovascular accident a few months ago. His wife is able to select and provide sufficient nutritious food for her husband.

Scale 9    Vulnerability
Scale 2    Availability

*A little baby girl* who is living in a drought area of Africa and is too weak to suck. Her mother is so malnourished that she has no milk. Water and food in this area is only available in small amounts infrequently.

Scale 10    Vulnerability
Scale 10    Availability

**Figure 4.2** *Completed chart to illustrate the interrelationships of clean water and nutritious food and the vulnerability of the individual*

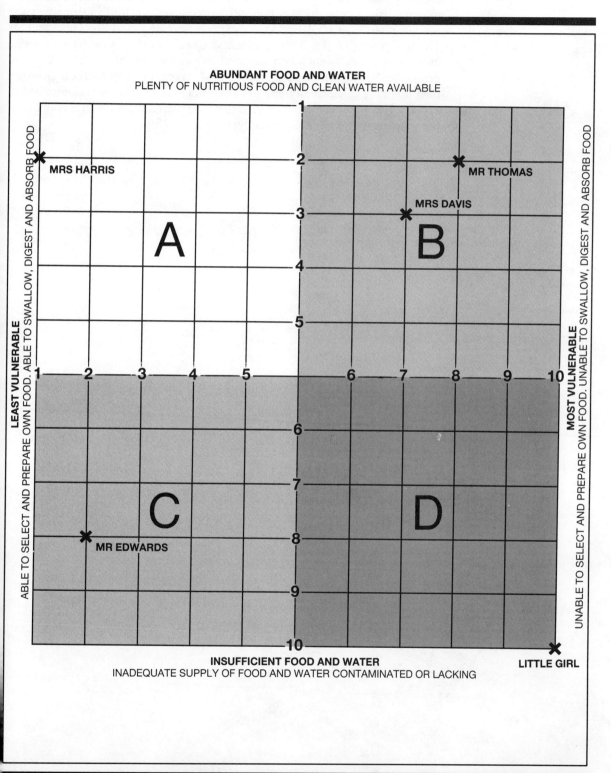

From the completed chart, *Figure 4.2*, you can see into which sections the different individuals fit. Mrs Harris is in Section A: this section illustrates minimal risk of difficulty in eating and drinking as she is fully independent and has adequate food available. Mr Edwards in Section C and Mrs Davis and Mr Thomas in Section B are all at some risk of developing problems with eating and drinking due to their own vulnerability or the lack of available food and drink. The baby girl in Section D is obviously at considerable risk both from her own inherent vulnerability and her environment. The measures described in *Figures 4.3, 4.4* and *4.5* can be considered to help reduce the vulnerability of the individual and minimise the effects of lack of food.

**Figure 4.3**  *Factors that can assist in providing clean water and adequate food*

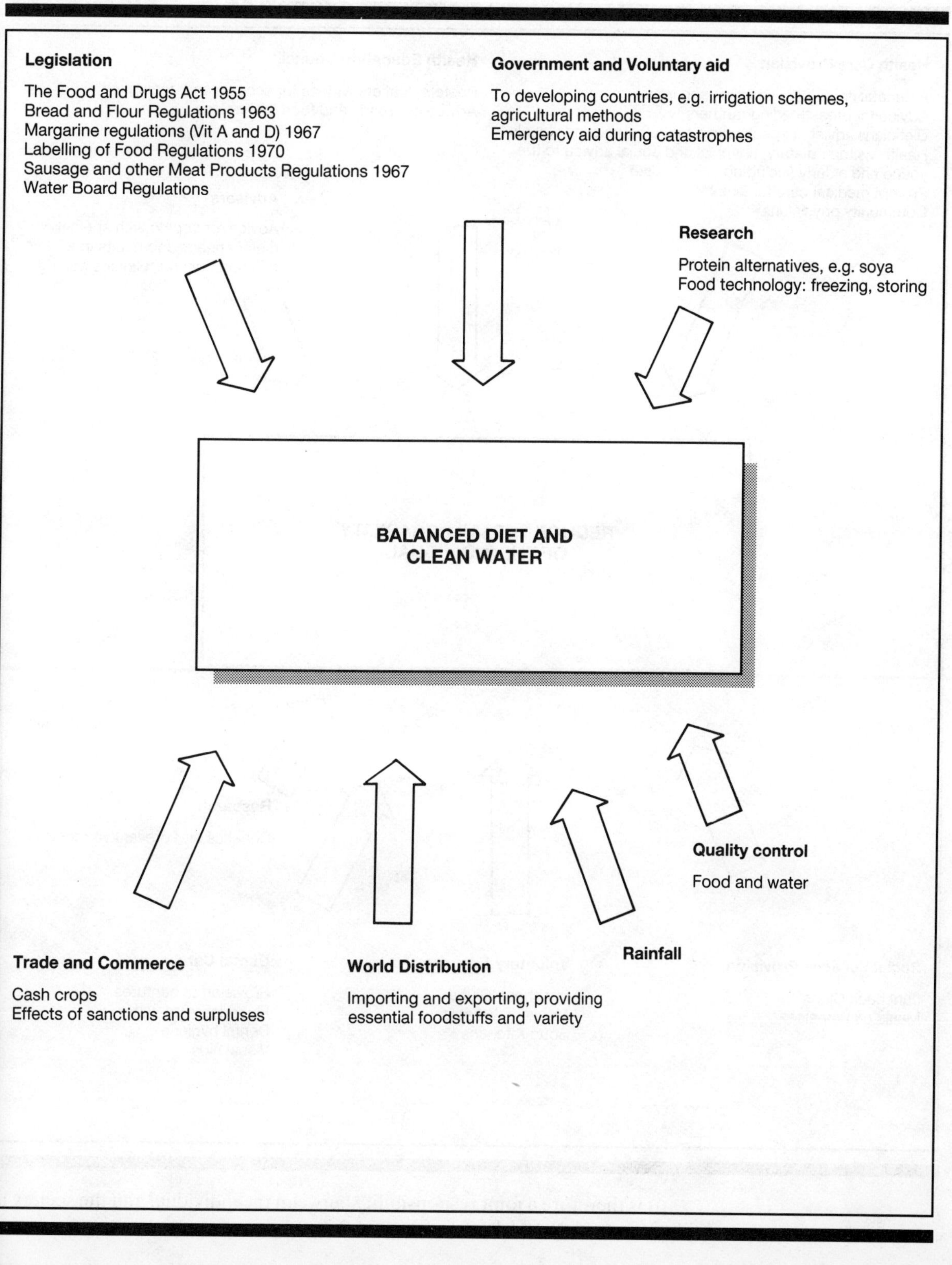

**Legislation**

The Food and Drugs Act 1955
Bread and Flour Regulations 1963
Margarine regulations (Vit A and D) 1967
Labelling of Food Regulations 1970
Sausage and other Meat Products Regulations 1967
Water Board Regulations

**Government and Voluntary aid**

To developing countries, e.g. irrigation schemes,
agricultural methods
Emergency aid during catastrophes

**Research**

Protein alternatives, e.g. soya
Food technology: freezing, storing

**BALANCED DIET AND
CLEAN WATER**

**Quality control**

Food and water

**Trade and Commerce**

Cash crops
Effects of sanctions and surpluses

**World Distribution**

Importing and exporting, providing
essential foodstuffs and variety

**Rainfall**

**Figure 4.4**   *Factors that can reduce the vulnerability of the individual*

**Health Care Provision**

Antenatal care: extra vitamins and iron
Advice for breastfeeding mothers
Dieticians advising special diets for vulnerable individuals
Health visitors: dietary, financial and social advice to the
young and elderly (including child abuse)
Prompt medical care for illness
Community physicians

**Health Education Council**

Posters, leaflets, videos for schools and general public
Advice on trends and food technology

**Advisors**

Advice for coping with special
dietary needs and habits in a
different cultural/religious setting

**REDUCE THE VULNERABILITY
OF THE INDIVIDUAL**

**Research**

Genetics and preventive medicine

**Social Services Provision**

Luncheon Clubs
Meals on Wheels

**Voluntary Services**

Luncheon Clubs
Meals on Wheels
Soup Kitchens

**Dental Care**

Provision of dentures
Fluoridation of water
Dental hygiene
Visual aids

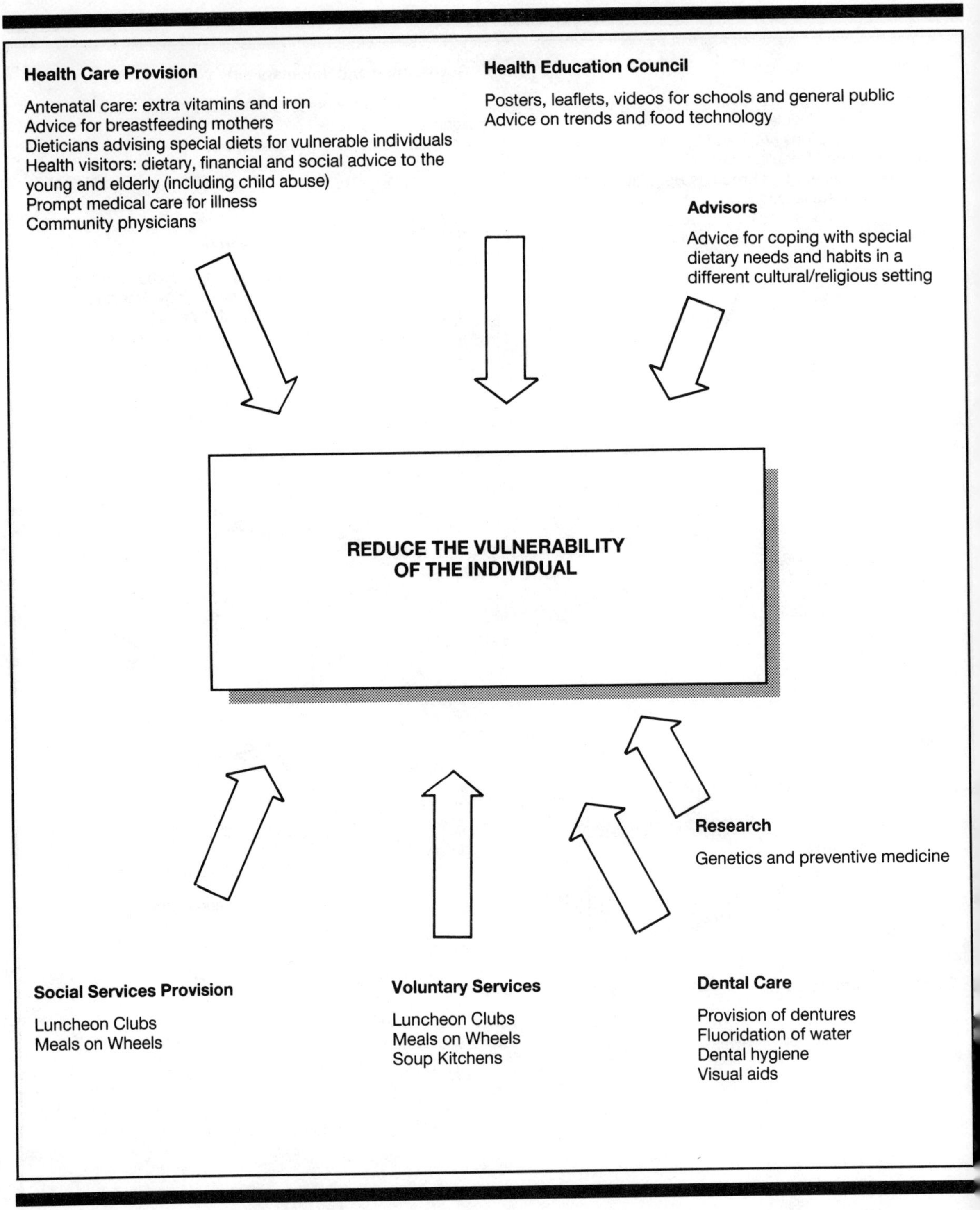

It is therefore a joint responsibility between the individual and the society h
lives in to reduce risk and make provision.

# PSYCHOLOGICAL FACTORS AFFECTING EATING AND DRINKING

**Figure 4.5**    *Some psychological factors affecting eating and drinking*

**Over activity/excitement**

An appetite can reduce or lead to rapid or slow eating

**Previous associations and experiences**

Can lead to dislikes, avoidance in certain foods, e.g. offal. Development of food 'fads'.

**Fear, anxiety and boredom**

Can lead to under- or over-eating

**Child rearing practices**

The use of food as punishment or reward. Attention seeking behaviour by withholding swallowing

**EATING AND DRINKING**

**Self-gratification**

As a substitute for company or used to enhance social acceptance, e.g. giving gifts, providing celebratory meals and functions

**Changes in biorhythms**

For example, in shift and night workers, meals taken at unfamiliar times and out of normal social setting

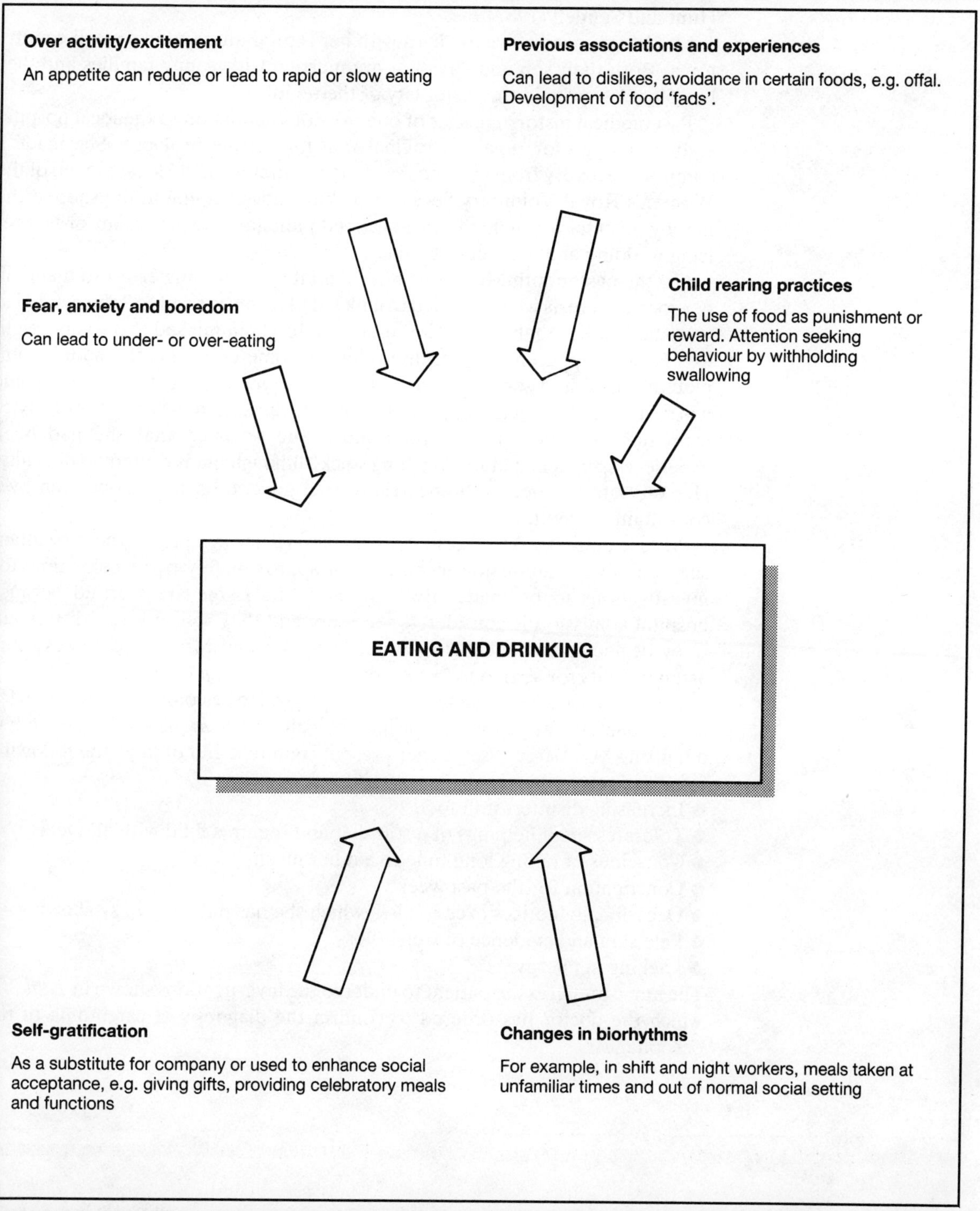

## PATIENT HISTORY

We would now like to consider a patient who has difficulty in eating and drinking. While you are reading Mrs Large's history it is important to bear in mind her vulnerability in relation to availability of adequate food. See also Hunt and Sendell (1987).

Mrs Large, aged 68 years, lives with her retired husband in a small country town. Both their son and daughter are married with young families and they live 50 miles away in the major city of the region.

Past medical history consists of one previous admission to the local hospital eight years ago for repair of vaginal wall for uterine prolapse. She made a complete recovery from this and resumed her interest in the local branch of the Women's Royal Voluntary Service which includes helping in the shop at the nearby hospital for mentally handicapped patients. She also takes orders for icing wedding and anniversary cakes.

For the past month Mrs Large has found it an increasing effort to maintain her social interests which seemed to make her feel more tired and she needed to go to bed earlier than usual. Her interest in food diminished and some weight loss became apparent. She realised that on some occasions she hadn't completed a meal and seemed to need to drink more while eating. She became worried about herself after regurgitating food during a meal and sought advice from her local doctor. On questioning, she revealed that she had been experiencing a feeling of food 'getting stuck' although fluids caused no difficulty. Her GP referred her to the nearest district general hospital to be seen by a consultant surgeon.

After examining Mrs Large and discussing her symptoms the consultant surgeon advises admission to hospital in approximately two weeks' time for investigations to be made. Both Mr and Mrs Large are worried because hospital admission is considered necessary and they return home distressed. They decide to contact their son and daughter and Mrs Large makes some arrangements for someone to take over her immediate commitments.

On admission Mrs Large seems almost pleased to be coming into hospital for some relief of her now increasing difficulty with swallowing. The nurse admitting Mrs Large assesses her present condition and obtains the following information:

- Increasing disinterest in food.
- Tolerates small helpings of a soft diet and requires fluid with all meals.
- Conscious of taking long time to eat her meal.
- Constipation for the past week.
- Occasionally notices excess saliva which she has difficulty in swallowing.
- Pale skin and evidence of weight loss.
- Lacking in energy.

The nurse prepares the patient to undergo the investigations shown in *Table 4.* which the doctor has ordered to confirm the diagnosis of carcinoma of the oesophagus.

*Table 4.1    Investigations (see Hunt and Sendell  1987)*

| Investigation | Abnormal findings |
| --- | --- |
| Blood tests for:<br>  Haemoglobin<br>  Electrolytes | Haemoglobin 9 g/100 ml<br>Normal |
| Fibre-optic endoscopy and biopsy | Abnormal mucous lining in middle third of oesophagus with evidence of infiltration to muscle layer causing stenosis<br><br>Biopsy: infiltrating carcinoma |
| Chest x-ray | No abnormal findings |

On confirmation of the diagnosis, Mrs Large is referred to the local consultant radiotherapist.

## EXPLANATION OF CLINICAL FEATURES

The clinical features of the disease affecting Mrs Large's alimentary system are explained in *Table 4.2*.

*Table 4.2  Abnormal physiology and clinical features*

| Normal physiology | Abnormal physiology | Clinical features |
|---|---|---|
| The oesophagus passes food by peristalsis from the mouth to the stomach. There is usually a 1–2 second delay at the lower end of the oesophagus (at the cardiac sphincter) | Lumen of oesophagus blocked at its lower end by a carcinoma. Peristalsis is unable to overcome the obstruction and food and fluids accumulate proximal to the obstruction | As the lumen of the oesophagus becomes obstructed Mrs Large finds it takes longer to eat a meal and progressively only copes with small amounts of softer foods. Anything not well chewed seems to get stuck. Eventually no solid food can pass the obstruction and regurgitation occurs |
| Saliva is produced in response to thinking about food, smelling, seeing and tasting food. It is swallowed mixed with the food and starts the digestion of cooked starches by chemical action. Water content of the saliva is reabsorbed into the bloodstream from the stomach and intestines | Saliva is still produced up to 1 litre a day and is swallowed mixed with food. As the obstruction increases the food/saliva mixture is regurgitated. Chemical activity is reduced on starches. Risk of dehydration as saliva is produced and lost | Conscious of the saliva in her mouth which she sometimes has to spit out |
| Food/saliva mixture enter the stomach and small intestines where it is digested, absorbed and utilised by the body for the production of heat and energy, growth and repair | Insufficient nutrients available in the stomach and small intestine for absorption and utilisation by the body to maintain its normal functioning | Lack of energy due to lack of calories. Pale skin due to anaemia from lack of iron. Weight loss due to lack of calories from carbohydrates, proteins and fats |
| The large colon collects the residue of digestion, reabsorbs water and excretes waste products as faeces at intervals | Reduced amounts of residue are received by the colon, water reabsorption continues | Lack of bulk in the faeces resulting in reduced excretion of faeces and constipation |

## EFFECTS OF DIFFICULTY WITH EATING AND DRINKING ON LIVING ACTIVITIES

Eating and drinking is normally carried out with pleasure, satisfying the nutritional and fluid needs of the body and carried out in such a way that i socially acceptable within the individual's cultural environment. It permit the individual to meet physiological, security, achievement and self-fulfilmen needs. If a person has difficulty in eating and drinking the living activitie could be affected.

### Difficulty with Eating and Drinking

1. *Breathing*
   Not affected.

2. *Eating and Drinking*
   A longer time is taken to eat as difficulty increases. Increasingly become socially unacceptable. Loss of pleasure and independence.

3. *Eliminating*
   Altered due to lack of bulk in diet. Reduced fluid output as intak decreases.

4. *Sleeping and Resting*
Could be disturbed as hunger and thirst increases. Could be disturbed due to difficulty in swallowing saliva.

5. *Moving*
Lack of energy due to insufficient nutrients.

6. *Maintaining Body Temperature*
Lack of production of heat causes body temperature to lower.

7. *Keeping the Body Clean*
May require assistance due to lack of energy from insufficient nutrients. Skin becomes dry and flaking and prone to infection due to poor hydration and poor regeneration of skin cells.

8. *Dressing Suitably*
Loss of heat production increases the need for warmer clothes. Loss of weight results in clothes becoming ill fitting.

9. *Avoiding Dangers and Injuries*
Delayed healing due to poor nutritional state. Prone to accident and injury because of reduced energy levels.

10. *Communicating*
Loss of social contact from the sociable aspects of eating and drinking. Diminished energy capacity limits social interaction.

11. *Worshipping*
Lack of energy to attend formal gatherings.

12. *Working*
May be unable to follow normal work.

13. *Participating in Recreation*
Dependent on physical capability, change may be necessary.

14. *Learning to Satisfy Curiosity*
May become increasingly questioning about his/her condition or may be so concerned with the problem that curiosity is dulled.

## A METHOD TO ASSIST YOU IN ASSESSING MRS LARGE

As in Chapter 3 an assessment sheet (*Figure 4.6*) now follows for which we would like you to complete the top section only at this stage, i.e. give consideration to the conditions always present that affect her basic needs. Circle the appropriate features relating to Mrs Large, i.e. age, temperament, social setting, capabilities and physiological disturbances. This will assist you to complete a personal profile of Mrs Large.

**Figure 4.6**   *A patient profile to assist in assessing patients and the development of a problem-solving approach to care*

Name _____ Mrs Large _____ No. _____

Address _____

Circle any features that are present in your patient in each of the five columns. Remember that more than one is possible in most of the columns

Section A    1. Starting with the age column, take your selected condition and consider each of the 14 functions requiring assistance and tick in the box(es) those appropriate to your patient's needs, e.g. an elderly patient may require assistance with 2, 3 and 5

Section B    2. Repeat the same procedure with subsequent columns

**(A)  Conditions always present that affect basic needs**

| *Age* | *Temperament* | *Social/Cultural* | *Physical/Intellectual Capacity* | **Physiological disturbances** |
|---|---|---|---|---|
| Newborn | Emotional state | Member of a family | Normal weight | 1. Fluid and electrolyte imbalance |
| Child | or passing mode: | unit with friends | Over-weight | 2. Oxygen want |
| Adolescent | (a) normal | and status | Under-weight | 3. Shock |
| Adult | (b) euphoric, | A person relatively | Normal mentality | 4. Consciousness |
| Middle aged | hyperactive | alone | Gifted mentality | 5. Local injury/ disease |
| Elderly | (c) anxious, fearful, | Maladjusted | Normal sense of: | 6. Metabolism |
| Aged | agitated, | Destitute | hearing | 7. Seeing, hearing, smell and touch |
| | hysterical | Smoker | sight | 8. Communicable conditions |
| | (d) depressed/ | Drinker | equilibrium | 9. Immobilisation: disease/treatment |
| | hypoactive | | touch | |
| | | | Loss of sense of: | |
| | | | hearing | |
| | | | sight | |
| | | | equilibrium | |
| | | | touch | |
| | | | Normal motor power | |
| | | | Loss of motor power | |

**(B)**

| **Functions requiring assistance** | *Age* | *Temperament* | *Social/Cultural* | *Physical/Intellectual Capacity* | *Physiological Disturbance* |
|---|---|---|---|---|---|
| 1. Breathing | | | | | |
| 2. Eating or drinking | | | | | |
| 3. Elimination | | | | | |
| 4. Sleep or rest | | | | | |
| 5. Movement | | | | | |
| 6. Maintenance of body temperature | | | | | |
| 7. Keeping body clean | | | | | |
| 8. Dressing suitably | | | | | |
| 9. Avoiding dangers and injury | | | | | |
| 10. Communication | | | | | |
| 11. Worship | | | | | |
| 12. Work | | | | | |
| 13. Participation in recreation | | | | | |
| 14. Learning to satisfy curiosity | | | | | |

Now use this information to decide which of her total needs (physiological, security, achievement and self-fulfilment) may be altered for her as an individual at this time. As a guide refer to the sample profiles in Section 1, Chapter 2, numbers 9 and 15 and decide how Mrs Large is different. Check your ideas with our completed profile shown in *Figure 4.7*.

**Figure 4.7**   *Profile for Mrs Large*

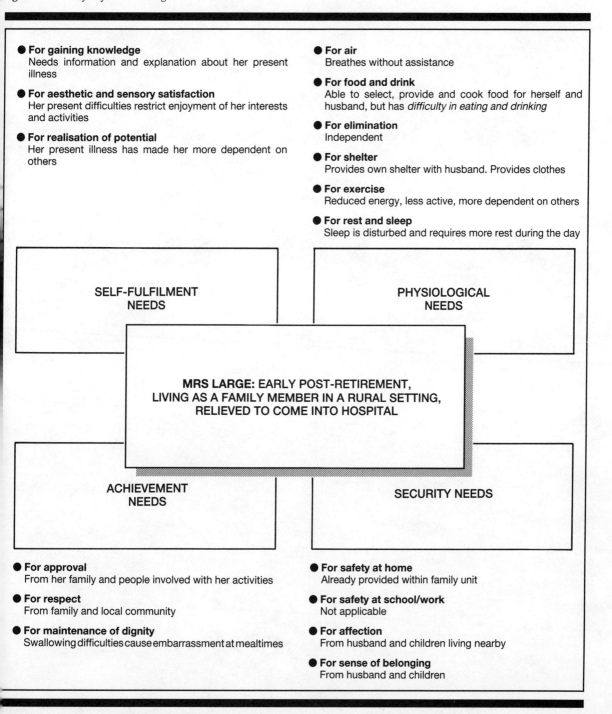

**For gaining knowledge**
Needs information and explanation about her present illness

**For aesthetic and sensory satisfaction**
Her present difficulties restrict enjoyment of her interests and activities

**For realisation of potential**
Her present illness has made her more dependent on others

**For air**
Breathes without assistance

**For food and drink**
Able to select, provide and cook food for herself and husband, but has *difficulty in eating and drinking*

**For elimination**
Independent

**For shelter**
Provides own shelter with husband. Provides clothes

**For exercise**
Reduced energy, less active, more dependent on others

**For rest and sleep**
Sleep is disturbed and requires more rest during the day

SELF-FULFILMENT NEEDS

PHYSIOLOGICAL NEEDS

**MRS LARGE:** EARLY POST-RETIREMENT, LIVING AS A FAMILY MEMBER IN A RURAL SETTING, RELIEVED TO COME INTO HOSPITAL

ACHIEVEMENT NEEDS

SECURITY NEEDS

**For approval**
From her family and people involved with her activities

**For respect**
From family and local community

**For maintenance of dignity**
Swallowing difficulties cause embarrassment at mealtimes

**For safety at home**
Already provided within family unit

**For safety at school/work**
Not applicable

**For affection**
From husband and children living nearby

**For sense of belonging**
From husband and children

You are now in a position to complete the lower section of the assessment sheet (*Figure 4.6*). Starting with the age column take your selected feature (previously circled) and consider each of the 14 functions requiring assistance and tick in the boxes those appropriate to Mrs Large's needs. Repeat the same procedure with the subsequent columns. Check your completed assessment sheet with the one that follows, *Figure 4.8*.

**Figure 4.8** *A patient profile to assist in assessing patients and the development of a problem-solving approach to care*

Name _____ Mrs Large _____ No. _____

Address _____

Circle any features that are present in your patient in each of the five columns.
Remember that more than one is possible in most of the columns

Section A   1. Starting with the age column, take your selected condition and consider each of the 14 functions requiring assistance and tick in the box(es) those appropriate to your patient's needs, e.g. an elderly patient may require assistance with 2, 3 and 5

Section B   2. Repeat the same procedure with subsequent columns

**(A) Conditions always present that affect basic needs**　　　　**Physiological disturbances**

| Age | Temperament | Social/Cultural | Physical/Intellectual Capacity | Physiological disturbances |
|---|---|---|---|---|
| Newborn | Emotional state | Member of a family | Capacity | 1. Fluid and electrolyte imbalance |
| Child | or passing mode: | unit with friends | Normal weight | 2. Oxygen want |
| Adolescent | (a) normal | and status | Over-weight | 3. Shock |
| Adult | (b) euphoric, | A person relatively | Under-weight | 4. Consciousness |
| Middle aged | hyperactive | alone | Normal mentality | 5. Local injury/disease |
| Elderly | (c) anxious, fearful, | Maladjusted | Gifted mentality | 6. Metabolism |
| Aged | agitated, hysterical | Destitute | Normal sense of: hearing sight equilibrium touch | 7. Seeing, hearing, smell and touch |
| | (d) depressed/hypoactive | Smoker Drinker | Loss of sense of: hearing sight equilibrium touch | 8. Communicable conditions |
| | | | Normal motor power Loss of motor power | 9. Immobilisation: disease/treatment |

**(B)**

| Functions requiring assistance | Age | Temperament | Social/Cultural | Physical/Intellectual Capacity | Physiological Disturbance |
|---|---|---|---|---|---|
| 1. Breathing | | | | | |
| 2. Eating or drinking | | | | | ✓ |
| 3. Elimination | | | | | ✓ |
| 4. Sleep or rest | | | | | ✓ |
| 5. Movement | | | | | ✓ |
| 6. Maintenance of body temperature | | | | | likely |
| 7. Keeping body clean | | | | | ✓ |
| 8. Dressing suitably | | | | | ✓ |
| 9. Avoiding dangers and injury | | | | | ✓ |
| 10. Communication | | | | | ✓ |
| 11. Worship | | | | | ✓ |
| 12. Work | | | | | no longer able |
| 13. Participation in recreation | | | | | no longer able |
| 14. Learning to satisfy curiosity | | | | | ✓ |

Now you know that Mrs Large's age, temperament, social setting, mental and physical capacities enable her to meet her physiological, security, achievement and self-fulfilment needs independently. Therefore the functions requiring assistance are wholly as a result of her physiological disturbance. From this you can develop a problem-solving approach to care.

## SELECTING NURSING ACTIONS TO ASSIST A PATIENT WITH DIFFICULTY IN EATING AND DRINKING

The main problem being discussed in this chapter is *difficulty in eating and drinking*. We would now like you to choose from the List of Nursing Actions shown in *Table 4.3* those appropriate for Mrs Large, by putting a tick in the Yes column if you think the action is appropriate, or in the No column if you think the action is inappropriate or dangerous, or in the Maybe column if you think the action is possible. Whatever your decision give an explanation for each of your choices and when you have completed this compare your decisions and explanations with those given on pages 96 to 99.

*Table 4.3   Nursing action to assist a patient with difficulty in eating and drinking*

| Nursing actions | Yes | No | Maybe | Reason for choice |
|---|---|---|---|---|
| **Part 1   Breathing** | | | | |
| 1. Provide suction apparatus at bedside | | | | |
| 2. Support patient by pillows | | | | |
| 3. Emergency tracheostomy set available | | | | |
| **Part 2   Eating and Drinking** | | | | |
| 1. Provide normal diet | | | | |
| 2. Provide soft diet | | | | |
| 3. Provide fluid diet | | | | |
| 4. Assist in provision of intravenous feeding | | | | |
| 5. Provide gastrostomy feeding | | | | |
| 6. Provide nasogastric feeding | | | | |
| 7. Give two large meals a day | | | | |
| 8. Give small frequent meals during the day | | | | |
| 9. Give small frequent meals day and night | | | | |
| 10. Help the patient to eat whatever she is able to manage | | | | |
| 11. Give bulky foods to dilate the oesophagus | | | | |

*Table 4.3 Continued*

| Nursing actions | Yes | No | Maybe | Reason for choice |
|---|---|---|---|---|
| **Part 2   Eating and Drinking (continued)** | | | | |
| 12. Give hourly high protein and carbohydrate drinks | | | | |
| 13. Give clear fluids only | | | | |
| 14. Give carbonated drinks | | | | |
| 15. Give high protein diet with extra meat | | | | |
| 16. Encourage to sit at table with others at meal-times | | | | |
| 17. Provide absolute privacy to eat and drink | | | | |
| 18. Provide a bib | | | | |
| 19. Encourage staff in providing a sensitive and patient approach | | | | |
| 20. Encourage patient to complete meals in allotted time | | | | |
| 21. Ensure patient finishes all that is offered | | | | |
| 22. Encourage patient to eat chocolates and sweets | | | | |
| 23. Offer drinks with food | | | | |
| **Part 3   Eliminating** | | | | |
| 1. Give suppositories | | | | |
| 2. Provide high fibre diet | | | | |
| 3. Give an enema | | | | |
| 4. Give an aperient | | | | |
| 5. Allow patient to go to the toilet as required | | | | |
| 6. Provide commode during day | | | | |
| 7. Provide commode at night | | | | |
| 8. Offer bedpans as required | | | | |
| **Part 4   Sleeping and Resting** | | | | |
| 1. Provide high protein drinks during the night if patient is hungry | | | | |
| 2. Offer night sedation | | | | |

*Table 4.3    Continued*

| Nursing actions | Yes | No | Maybe | Reason for choice |
|---|---|---|---|---|
| **Part 4   Sleeping and Resting (continued)** | | | | |
| 3. Offer warm drink on settling at night | | | | |
| 4. Encourage the patient to sleep sitting up well supported on pillows | | | | |
| 5. Encourage the patient to have rest periods during the day | | | | |
| 6. Discourage the patient from taking cat naps during the day | | | | |
| **Part 5   Moving** | | | | |
| 1. Keep the patient at complete rest | | | | |
| 2. Encourage exercise | | | | |
| 3. Sit in easy chair | | | | |
| 4. Assist in repositioning in bed | | | | |
| 5. Provide sheepskin | | | | |
| 6. Provide ripple bed | | | | |
| 7. Provide hoist | | | | |
| 8. Offer assistance and provide supervision if patient is weak or dizzy | | | | |
| **Part 6   Maintaining Body Temperature** | | | | |
| 1. Provide plenty of blankets | | | | |
| 2. Provide warm clothing | | | | |
| 3. Provide light bed clothes | | | | |
| 4. Ensure adequate ventilation | | | | |
| 5. Give hot-water bottle | | | | |
| **Part 7   Keeping Body Clean** | | | | |
| 1. Give daily bed bath | | | | |
| 2. Assist patient with washing in bed | | | | |
| 3. Assist patient with washing in the bathroom | | | | |
| 4. Encourage patient to bath herself | | | | |

*Table 4.3    Continued*

| Nursing actions | Yes | No | Maybe | Reason for choice |
|---|---|---|---|---|
| **Part 7    Keeping Body Clean (continued)** | | | | |
| 5. Assist patient to brush hair | | | | |
| 6. Offer antiseptic mouthwashes after meals | | | | |
| 7. Give oral toilet | | | | |
| 8. Provide plenty of tissues and disposal bag | | | | |
| **Part 8    Dressing Suitably** | | | | |
| 1. Provide hospital nightdress | | | | |
| 2. Encourage use of own nightdress | | | | |
| 3. Encourage patient to dress normally during day | | | | |
| **Part 9    Avoiding Dangers and Injury** | | | | |
| 1. Ensure a member of staff is always in the ward while patient is eating | | | | |
| 2. Check ward floor is free of spillages | | | | |
| 3. Allow patient to prepare her own drinks as required | | | | |
| **Part 10    Communicating** | | | | |
| 1. Allocate a nurse to the patient | | | | |
| 2. Encourage husband to assist with care | | | | |
| 3. Encourage free visiting | | | | |
| 4. Discourage visitors during mealtimes | | | | |
| 5. Ensure messages from the family are delivered to the patient | | | | |
| 6. Give opportunity for exchange of information and explanation between staff, patient and relatives | | | | |
| 7. Provide opportunity for patient to meet and discuss progress with dietitian | | | | |
| 8. Report that the patient has been 'difficult' with her eating | | | | |
| 9. Tell the patient she must not think about her voluntary responsibilities until she is better | | | | |

*Table 4.3    Continued*

| Nursing actions | Yes | No | Maybe | Reason for choice |
|---|---|---|---|---|
| **Part 10   Communicating (continued)**<br><br>10. Take an interest in the patient's outside activities and hobbies | | | | |
| **Part 11   Worshipping**<br><br>1. Inform hospital chaplain<br><br>2. Inform patient's own chaplain of patient's admission<br><br>3. Ignore spiritual needs until patient is feeling better<br><br>4. Make provision for patient to attend hospital chapel | | | | |
| **Part 12   Working**<br><br>Patient is retired and not in permanent employment | | | | |
| **Part 13   Participating in Recreation**<br><br>1. Assist in choosing suitable diversional therapy<br><br>2. Encourage and show interest in patient's own activities<br><br>3. Encourage the patient in physical exercise to build up her strength | | | | |
| **Part 14   Learning to Satisfy Curiosity**<br><br>1. Keep patient and husband fully informed of her condition and progress<br><br>2. Tell the patient not to worry about food as correct diet will be supplied to her<br><br>3. Avoid discussing long-term expectations | | | | |

## EXPLANATION FOR CHOICE OF NURSING ACTIONS

### Part 1    Breathing

We hope you have ticked the Yes column for number 1. Because of Mr Large's difficulty in eating and drinking there is a potential danger of he choking. You may have ticked the Maybe column for numbers 2 and 3. I she is weak she may need support from pillows to make swallowing easier The emergency tracheostomy set should always be available for patients a risk.

*Part 2 Eating and Drinking*

We hope you have ticked the Yes column for numbers 8, 10, 19, 23. Small frequent meals with fluids will help to maintain her intake and will continue what she found helpful prior to admission. She needs a sensitive and supportive approach from the staff in order to make it possible for her to still remain in control of her intake.

You may have ticked the Maybe column for numbers 2, 3, 4, 5, 6, 9, 12, 14, 16, 17. The provision of soft, fluid diet or alternative methods of feeding will depend on Mrs Large's ability to eat and drink. Numbers 9 and 12 if she is able to eat and drink a little; by giving small frequent meals throughout the 24 hours and hourly high protein and carbohydrate drink it may be more possible to maintain adequate nutrition. Number 14: the effervescent effect of these drinks can help to keep the lumen of the oesophagus free of food debris and can be mixed with other fluids such as milk. Numbers 16 and 17: eating and drinking is normally a social activity and therefore could be an embarrassment to Mrs Large if she is having to eat slowly and with difficulty in front of others. The staff therefore need to be sensitive in assisting Mrs Large to either sit at a table with others for meals or provide privacy at mealtimes.

We hope you have ticked the No column for numbers 1, 7, 11, 13, 15, 18, 20, 21, 22. Because Mrs Large has an obstruction in her oesophagus she cannot manage a normal diet, and she has not been able to cope with large meals recently. Bulky foods will only get stuck and will have no effect on the degree of stenosis. Food would tend to accumulate proximal to the obstruction and cause regurgitation. Giving clear fluids only would not provide essential nutrients; equally trying to provide a high protein diet using meat is inappropriate as meat is particularly difficult to chew and swallow due to its texture. Number 22 is also not appropriate since Mrs Large needs to be encouraged to concentrate on eating and drinking essential foods. Number 18, providing a bib, is socially degrading as these are normally associated with children and babies. Numbers 20 and 21 would indicate insensitivity and failure to take account of Mrs Large's difficulties in eating and drinking and how she has attempted to cope with these difficulties. She should be given as much time as she needs in order to eat what she can manage.

*Part 3 Eliminating*

You could have ticked in the Yes column for numbers 1, 5 and 8. Mrs Large is constipated due to lack of bulk and fluid in the diet and may need suppositories. Numbers 5 and 8 depend on the amount of assistance that she may need, day and night. You could have ticked numbers 6 and 7 in the Maybe column for the same reason. Numbers 2, 3 and 5 should be ticked in the No column as she cannot swallow a high fibre diet and an enema or aperients are over-stimulating to the gastrointestinal tract.

*Part 4 Sleeping and Resting*

We hope you have ticked numbers 3, 4 and 5 in the Yes column. A warm drink at night on settling is relaxing, comforting, nutritious and helps to maintain fluid intake. By sitting Mrs Large upright to sleep it reduces pressure of the abdominal contents on the diaphragm and back pressure on the oesophagus. It can help to prevent disturbance by regurgitation during sleep.

You could have ticked the Maybe column for numbers 1 and 2. These can help to ensure adequate rest by either providing medication or reducing sleeplessness from hunger. Number 6 is not appropriate since Mrs Large needs as much rest as she can get throughout the 24 hours to conserve her energy.

### Part 5   Moving

We suggest that you should have ticked numbers 3 and 8 in the Yes column. Mrs Large needs to have the opportunity to move around but she may be quite weak and prefer to rest frequently in an easy chair. When up and about she needs to be offered assistance if she feels weak and dizzy. You could have ticked numbers 2, 4, 5 and 7 in the Maybe column. She may be depressed by her condition and needs encouragement to exercise according to her capabilities. However, if she is very weak she may be confined to bed in which case she may need a sheepskin and hoist and assistance with moving in bed as she is likely to be thin and lethargic and at risk of developing pressure sores and other complications of bed rest. Numbers 1 and 6 are inappropriate as complete rest would take away her independence and increase her risk. A ripple bed is unlikely to be needed at this time.

### Part 6   Maintaining Body Temperature

You should have ticked number 4 in the Yes column as this is a normal requirement. Numbers 1 and 2 should be ticked in the Maybe column because if Mrs Large has lost weight and is less able to generate heat she may need extra blankets and clothing. Numbers 3 and 5 should be ticked in the No column: light bedclothes are inappropriate and a hot-water bottle is a potential hazard in preparing and using.

### Part 7   Keeping Body Clean

In the Yes column you should have ticked numbers 3, 4, 6 and 8. Mrs Large is likely to require help and encouragement with washing and bathing. Antiseptic mouthwashes help to keep the oral cavity free of debris and infection and tissues should always be available for her to remove saliva and debris in a sociably acceptable manner if she is unable to swallow. Numbers 2, 5 and 7 may be necessary. Number 1 is not likely to be appropriate.

### Part 8   Dressing Suitably

You should have ticked numbers 2 and 3 in the Yes column. Using her own clothes and getting dressed during the day will help her sense of well-being and independence. Number 1 should be in the Maybe column since hospital clothes may be needed in an emergency, for example if she vomits.

### Part 9   Avoiding Dangers and Injury

You should have ticked numbers 1 and 2 in the Yes column and number 3 in the Maybe column. Mrs Large is at risk during mealtimes of inhaling regurgitated food and if she is weak she may not be alert to hazards such as wet floors, heavy kitchen equipment and using boiling water.

### Part 10   Communicating

You should have ticked the Yes column for numbers 1, 2, 3, 5, 6, 7 and 8. All these provide the opportunity for listening, talking and exchanging info mation about her fears, anxieties and feelings with all members of staff, husband and other family members.

Number 4 should be ticked in the Maybe column if Mrs Large prefers to have privacy during meals. Numbers 8 and 9 should be ticked in the No column. Patients should not be labelled 'difficult' as this can influence other staff, affect attitudes and develop the staff's biases and prejudices against them. A more objective view is needed to determine the possible causes of the patient's behaviour.

Number 9 is not appropriate. Mrs Large needs to have the opportunity to discuss her present concerns since these do not disappear just because she has been admitted to hospital.

### Part 11    Worshipping

Items 1, 2 and 4 could have been ticked in the Maybe column if and whichever the patient wishes. Number 3 should be in the No column; if acknowledged by the patient, spiritual needs should be met promptly.

### Part 12    Working

Mrs Large is retired and this section is not applicable.

### Part 13    Participating in Recreation

Numbers 1 and 2 should be in the Yes column. Encouragement and support is required to help patient to choose a suitable diversional activity. Number 3 should be No. Mrs Large needs to conserve her strength and energy at this time.

### Part 14    Learning to Satisfy Curiosity

You should have ticked number 1 in the Yes column to alleviate fear of the unknown. Numbers 2 and 3 should be in the No column: Mrs Large has a right to be concerned about her diet and her prognosis and these should be fully discussed with her as required.

### CHOOSING PRIORITIES IN NURSING ACTIONS

This is the list of Henderson's components of basic nursing care (Henderson, 1969) which we have used in Parts 1–14.

Table 4.4    Priorities in nursing actions

| Part | Insert your choice of priority nos. 1–14 |
|---|---|
| 1. Breathing | |
| 2. Eating and drinking | |
| 3. Eliminating | |
| 4. Sleeping and resting | |
| 5. Moving | |
| 6. Maintaining body temperature | |

*Table 4.4  Continued*

|  |  |
|---|---|
| 7.  Keeping body clean |  |
| 8.  Dressing suitably |  |
| 9.  Avoiding dangers and injury |  |
| 10.  Communicating |  |
| 11.  Worshipping |  |
| 12.  Working |  |
| 13.  Participating in recreation |  |
| 14.  Learning to satisfy curiosity |  |

In Table 4.4 we would now like you to number each of the components you would consider in order of priority for Mrs Large while she has difficulty in eating and drinking.

Use Table 4.5 to help you to decide on your actions in planning care.

*Table 4.5  Necessary actions in planning and providing nursing care*

|  | Please refer to headings of columns on Plan of Care |
|---|---|
| ● Decide on appropriate care | Yes |
| ● Decide on potential care | Maybe |
| ● Decide on what to do first, second and third, etc | Priority choice |
| ● Decide which observations or measurements are needed to monitor patient's progress adequately | Measurements |
| ● Select realistic outcomes | Short-term goals |
| ● Decide when to review results of nursing actions | Review period |
| ● Give opportunity for stating results of evaluation and possible alteration of short-term goals and review period | Evaluation criteria |

You can check your decisions with the plan shown in *Table 4.6*. As you can see we consider Part 2 Eating and Drinking as the first priority, with Part 1 Breathing and Part 9 Avoiding Dangers and Injury as joint second priorities. Check your subsequent sequence with *Table 4.6*. Don't be surprised if you find some differences of opinions, as long as you can justify your decision without jeopardizing your patient's safety and well-being.

## IDENTIFICATION OF CRITERIA OF PROGRESS

You should now read carefully the plan shown in *Table 4.6* for identifying criteria for progress.

*Table 4.6 Plan of care for progress*

| Nursing actions to assist a patient with difficulty in eating and drinking | Yes | Maybe | Priority Choice | Measurements | Short-term goals | Review period | Evaluation Criteria Have short-term goals been met? |
|---|---|---|---|---|---|---|---|
| **Part 2 Eating and Drinking** | | | | Record: (a) How much food and fluids is eaten and drunk | (a), (b), (c), (d) Intake of 2 litres of fluid and 1500 calories in 24 hours | | (a), (b), (d) Has managed to drink 2 litres of fluid and consumed 1700 calories of soft foods only and high protein drinks |
| 2. Provide soft diet | | ✓ | | | | | |
| 3. Provide fluid diet | | ✓ | | (b) Frequency of taking food and drink | Not feeling hungry | | |
| 4. Assist in provision of intravenous feeding | | ✓ | | | | | |
| 5. Provide gastrostomy feeding | | ✓ | | (c) When she feels hunger | | 8-hourly | (c) Not hungry in daytime |
| | | | | (d) Type of intake: likes and dislikes | | | |
| 6. Provide nasogastric feeding | | ✓ | | (e) Weight | (e) Maintain present weight and possibly gain weight | Every 48 hours | (e) Stable |
| 8. Give small frequent meals during the day | ✓ | | | (f) Amount of regurgitated food and saliva | (f) Minimise the frequency and amount | 24-hourly | (f) Reduced in amount and frequency |
| 9. Give small frequent meals day and night | | ✓ | | (g) Take note of any distress or anxiety regarding eating with others | (g) Able to eat and drink without distress | At meal-times | (g) Prefers to take time and eat alone or with husband |
| 10. Help the patient to eat whatever she is able to manage | ✓ | | F I R S T | *Note*: If artificial feeding is required then the following measurements are necessary: | | | |
| 12. Give hourly high protein and carbohydrate drinks | | ✓ | | rate of administration | Same as (a)–(f) above | 24-hourly | Not needed |
| 14. Give carbonated drinks | | ✓ | | nature and amount of feed | | | |
| 16. Encourage patient to sit at table with others at mealtimes | | ✓ | | state of patency of tubes | | | |
| 17. Provide absolute privacy to eat and drink | | ✓ | | state of site, e.g. nose, abdominal wall, vein | | | |
| 19. Encourage staff in providing a sensitive and patient approach | ✓ | | | | | | |
| 23. Offer drinks with food | ✓ | | | | | | |

*Table 4.6    Continued*

| Nursing actions to assist a patient with difficulty in eating and drinking | Yes | Maybe | Priority Choice | Measurements | Short-term goals | Review period | Evaluation Criteria Have short-term goals been met? |
|---|---|---|---|---|---|---|---|
| **Part 1   Breathing**<br><br>1. Provide suction apparatus at bedside | ✓ | | | Note:<br>(a) Coughing<br>Cyanosis<br>Respiratory distress | (a) Safeguard against inhalation of food or saliva | At meal-times | (a) Has strong cough reflex, has not had any episodes of choking |
| 2. Support patient by pillows | | ✓ | | | | | |
| 3. Emergency tracheostomy set available | | ✓ | SECOND | | | | |
| **Part 9   Avoiding Dangers and Injury**<br><br>1. Ensure a member of staff is always in the ward while patient is eating | ✓ | | | (b) Prompt attention to spillages | (b) Prevent accidental injury | When required | (b) No accidents or incidents |
| 2. Check ward floor is free of spillages | ✓ | | | | | | |
| 3. Allow patient to prepare her own drinks as required | | ✓ | | | | | |
| **Part 10 Communicating**<br><br>1. Allocate a nurse to the patient | ✓ | | | Note:<br>levels of anxiety/ frustration from patient, relatives and staff | Mrs and Mr Large are confident in the care being given and feel able to relate to staff | On-going | Husband visits freely as he is retired, helps at mealtimes. Children have been in contact and dietician has visited for preliminary assessment. Medical staff have discussed progress and prognosis with Mrs and Mr Large |
| 2. Encourage husband to assist with care | ✓ | | | | | | |
| 3. Encourage free visiting | ✓ | | THIRD | | | | |
| 4. Discourage visitors during mealtimes | | ✓ | | | | | |
| 5. Ensure messages from the family are delivered to the patient | ✓ | | | | | | |
| 6. Give opportunity for exchange of information and explanation between staff, patient and relatives | ✓ | | | | | | |

*Table 4.6    Continued*

| Nursing actions to assist a patient with difficulty in eating and drinking | Yes | Maybe | Priority Choice | Measurements | Short-term goals | Review period | Evaluation Criteria Have short-term goals been met? |
|---|---|---|---|---|---|---|---|
| **Part 10 Communicating (continued)** | | | | | | | |
| 7. Provide opportunity for patient to meet and discuss progress with dietician | ✓ | | THIRD | | | | |
| 10. Take an interest in the patient's outside interests | ✓ | | | | | | |
| **Part 14   Learning to Satisfy Curiosity** | | | | | | | |
| 1. Keep patient and husband fully informed of her condition and progress | ✓ | | | | | | |
| **Part 4   Sleeping and Resting** | | | | Record: (a) Length of sleep | 6–7 hours undisturbed sleep/ rest | 24-hourly | Disturbed frequently, woken by excess saliva and hunger. Not fully refreshed, needs rest periods during the day |
| 1. Provide high protein drinks during the night if patient is hungry | | ✓ | | (b) Number of disturbances during the night | | | |
| 2. Offer night sedation | | ✓ | | (c) If disturbed what has wakened her | | | |
| 3. Offer warm drink on settling at night | ✓ | | FOURTH | (d) Whether she wakes refreshed | | | |
| 4. Encourage the patient to sleep sitting up, well supported on pillows | ✓ | | | Note whether night sedation required | | | |
| 5. Encourage the patient to have rest periods during the day | ✓ | | | | | | |
| **Part 5   Moving** | | | | Note: (a) Length of time she stays in bed | Able to be up and moving around for short periods with adequate rest | 24-hourly | Up and dressed for most of the day, resting for 2 hours after lunch |
| 2. Encourage exercise | | ✓ | | (b) Any episodes of weakness or dizziness | | | |
| 3. Sit in easy chair | ✓ | | | | | | |
| 4. Assist in repositioning in bed | | ✓ | | | | | |
| 5. Provide sheepskin | | ✓ | | | | | |
| 7. Provide hoist | | ✓ | | | | | |
| 8. Offer assistance and provide supervision if patient is weak or dizzy | ✓ | | | | | | |

*Table 4.6   Continued*

| Nursing actions to assist a patient with difficulty in eating and drinking | Yes | Maybe | Priority Choice | Measurements | Short-term goals | Review period | Evaluation Criteria Have short-term goals been met? |
|---|---|---|---|---|---|---|---|
| **Part 3   Eliminating** | | | FIFTH | (a) Measure and record urine output and regurgitation | (a) 24-hourly urine output of at least 1½ litres | 8-hourly | 24-hour total 1 litre of urine |
| 1. Give suppositories | ✓ | | | | | | |
| 5. Allow patient to go to the toilet as required | ✓ | | | (b) Note consistency and frequency of bowel action | (b) Restore normal bowel function | 24-hourly | No bowel action since admission |
| 6. Provide commode—daytime | | ✓ | | | | | |
| 7. Provide commode—night-time | | ✓ | | | | | |
| 8. Offer bedpans as required | ✓ | | | | | | |
| **Part 7   Keeping Body Clean** | | | SIXTH | Note: (a) patient's ability to cope with her own hygiene | (a) Maintain cleanliness during period of partial dependence | 24-hourly | (a) Manages to bath with a little help |
| 2. Assist patient with washing in bed | | ✓ | | | | | |
| 3. Assist patient with washing in the bathroom | ✓ | | | (b) State of skin, mouth, hair and nails | (b) Maintain good condition of skin, hair and nails | 8-hourly | (b) Skin intact and well cared for. Mouth moist, no cracks or abrasions |
| 4. Encourage patient to bath herself | ✓ | | | | | | |
| 5. Assist patient to brush hair | | ✓ | | | | | |
| 6. Offer antiseptic mouthwashes after meals | ✓ | | | (c) Amount of saliva produced | (c) Enable her to cope in a socially acceptable way | 8-hourly | (c) Not troublesome except at night |
| 7. Give oral toilet | | ✓ | | | | | |
| 8. Provide plenty of tissues and disposal bag | ✓ | | | | | | |
| **Part 6   Maintaining the Body Temperature** | | | SEVENTH | (a) Record body temperature daily (b) Check for adequate room temperature | Avoid chilling | 24-hourly | (a) (b) Body temperature within normal limits. Feels comfortable |
| 1. Provide plenty of blankets | | ✓ | | | | | |
| 2. Provide warm clothing | | ✓ | | | | | |
| 4. Ensure adequate ventilation | ✓ | | | | | | |

*Table 4.6   Continued*

| Nursing actions to assist a patient with difficulty in eating and drinking | Yes | Maybe | Priority Choice | Measurements | Short-term goals | Review period | Evaluation Criteria Have short-term goals been met? |
|---|---|---|---|---|---|---|---|
| **Part 8   Dressing Suitably**<br><br>1. Provide hospital nightdress<br><br>2. Encourage use of own nightdress<br><br>3. Encourage dressing normally during day | 2. ✓<br>3. ✓ | 1. ✓ | SEVENTH | Note her level of interest in obtaining and dressing in own clothes | Maintain her interest in her personal appearance | 24-hourly | Using her own clothes, day and night. Husband is replacing clothes as necessary |
| **Part 11   Worshipping**<br><br>1. Inform hospital chaplain<br><br>2. Inform patient's own chaplain of her admission<br><br>4. Make provision for patient to attend hospital chapel<br><br>**Part 13   Participating in Recreation**<br><br>1. Assist in choosing suitable diversional therapy<br><br>2. Encourage and show interest in patient's own activities | 1.(Part13) ✓<br>2.(Part13) ✓ | 1. ✓<br>2. ✓<br>4. ✓ | EIGHTH | Note Mrs Large's desire for spiritual help<br><br><br><br><br><br>Note how Mrs Large is occupying her day | Satisfaction of spiritual needs if necessary<br><br><br><br><br><br>To provide suitable stimulus if required | Within 48 hours<br><br><br><br><br><br>24-hourly | Link with own church continued. Would like to attend hospital chapel services<br><br><br><br><br><br>Has sufficient personal activities to keep her occupied: likes to read and write letters |

As mentioned in Chapter 3, by choosing appropriate review periods of patient's progress it is easy to identify which aspects of patient's progress have improved and therefore need less or different nursing assistance, those aspects which remain the same and therefore need continuation of nursing assistance and those that have deteriorated and need more and different assistance.

### Using Evaluation Criteria for Resetting Short-term Goals

We would like to suggest that you may like to reconsider Mrs Large's plan of care choosing appropriate nursing action, deciding new priorities and measurements and setting revised short-term goals, using our hypothetical evaluation criteria as your starting point. You should try to justify your thoughts in discussion with others, or in writing, to obtain feedback from your tutor or ward sister/nursing officer.

### IDENTIFICATION OF LONG-TERM GOALS

We would expect that after some form of surgery and/or radiotherapy the long-term goal for Mrs Large would be to return home, able to maintain her health and weight on as near normal a diet as possible. She should also be confident that professional help will be available as and when she requires it. When it has been determined that Mrs Large's treatment has been successful her long-term goals need to be identified to enable her to function at home with some assistance from others. If you remember the individual profiles numbers 9 and 15 in Section 1, Chapter 2, you can complete the outline shown in *Figure 4.9* to give a profile of Mrs Large which will indicate her *expected* level of independence for her age and social setting as a family member.

**Figure 4.9**  *Long-term goal profile for Mrs Large*

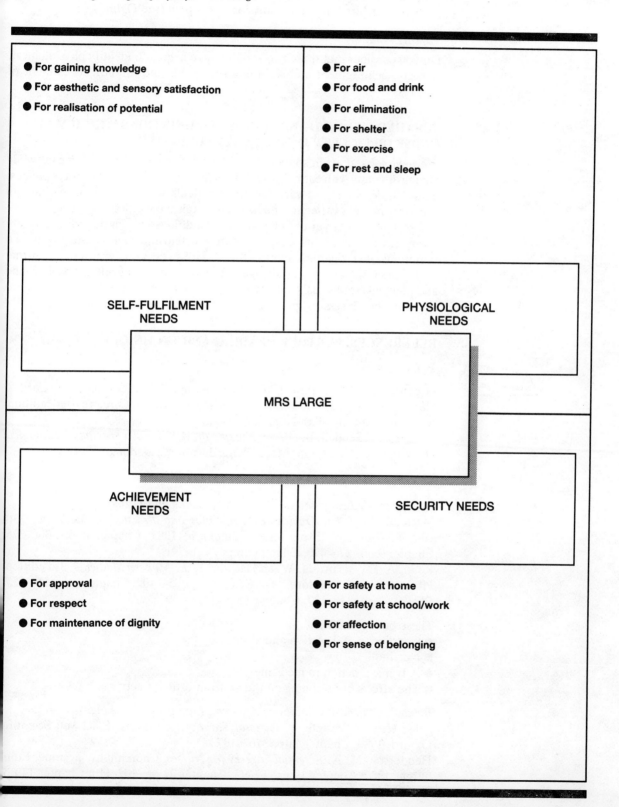

- For gaining knowledge
- For aesthetic and sensory satisfaction
- For realisation of potential

- For air
- For food and drink
- For elimination
- For shelter
- For exercise
- For rest and sleep

SELF-FULFILMENT
NEEDS

PHYSIOLOGICAL
NEEDS

MRS LARGE

ACHIEVEMENT
NEEDS

SECURITY NEEDS

- For approval
- For respect
- For maintenance of dignity

- For safety at home
- For safety at school/work
- For affection
- For sense of belonging

You may now like to compare this long-term goal profile with the one you prepared for Mrs Large on admission to hospital (see *Figure 4.7*).

### Talking Point

Do you consider that these two profiles have helped to identify physiological, security, achievement and self-fulfilment needs and to allow assessment of progress?

## FURTHER MEDICAL AND SURGICAL CONDITIONS WHICH MAY CAUSE DIFFICULTY IN EATING AND DRINKING

We have looked at, in some detail, Mrs Large's need for nursing care while having difficulty with eating and drinking due to obstruction of the oesophagus. You will be helping to care for other patients with difficulty in eating and drinking due to a variety of medical and surgical conditions.

References to a variety of common conditions causing this difficulty are given at the end of the chapter. You will find included causes, signs and symptoms, investigations and treatment. However, as before, remember that each patient will be of a certain age, temperament, social/cultural background and physical/intellectual capacity and all these factors must be taken fully into account when assessing, planning and reviewing the care required.

## REFERENCES, FURTHER READING AND TECHNIQUES

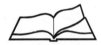

### References

Green, J. H. (1978). *Basic Clinical Physiology*, 3rd edition. OUP, Oxford.
Henderson, V. (1969). *Basic Principles of Nursing Care*, revised edition. International Council of Nurses, Geneva.
Hunt, P. and Sendell, B. (1987). *Nursing the Adult with a Specific Physiological Disturbance*. 2nd edition, Macmillan Education, London.

### Suggested Further Reading

*Related to Medical Conditions Affecting Eating and Drinking*
Macleod, J. (Ed.). *Davidson's Principles and Practice of Medicine*, 13th edition. Churchill Livingstone, Edinburgh, 1983: Chapter 8 pp. 308–375; Chapter 9 pp. 376–420; Chapter 16 pp. 781–791.
Read, A. E., Barritt, D. W. and Hewer, R. L. *Modern Medicine*, 3rd edition. Pitman Medical, London, 1984: Chapter 5 pp. 54–109; Chapter 6 pp. 110–117; Chapter 7 pp. 118–127; Chapter 15 pp. 254–260.

These books include:
● Conditions of digestion and absorption
● Nutrition
● Adverse reaction to medicines
● The effects of poisoning on the gastrointestinal tract

*Related to Surgical Conditions Affecting Eating and Drinking*
Ellis, H. and Wastell, C. *General Surgery for Nurses*. Blackwell Scientific Oxford, 1980, Chapter 11 pp. 162–197.
Henderson, M. A. *Essential Surgery for Nurses*. Churchill Livingstone, Edinburgh, 1980: Chapter 19 pp. 87–92; Chapter 22 pp. 102–110; Chapter 14 pp 50–53; Chapter 31 p. 166.

Horton, R. *General Surgery and the Nurse*. Hodder and Stoughton, London, 1983, Chapter 14 pp.101–138.

These books include:
● Trauma and conditions of jaw/mouth
● Surgery of oesophagus
● Peptic ulceration

### Pharmacology Related to Care of Patients with Difficulty in Eating and Drinking

You may wish to familiarise yourself with the medicines commonly used for patients with difficulty in eating and drinking, for example, antacids, muscle relaxants.

### Suggested Nursing Procedures / Guidelines for Nursing Practice

You may wish to familiarise yourself with your local policies and procedures/guidelines for nursing practice which may be applicable to a patient requiring assistance with difficulty in eating and drinking. Here is a suggested list:
● Artificial feeding
  gastrostomy
  nasogastric
  enteral and parenteral
● Endoscopic pre- and post-operative care
● Suppositories
● Suction equipment care and use
● Intravenous therapy
● Mouth care

# Chapter 5

# Eliminating

## NORMAL PHYSIOLOGY

Before proceeding we suggest you revise your knowledge of normal physiology of elimination by using the following references.

● Hunt and Sendell (1987). *Nursing the Adult with a Specific Physiological Disturbance*, 2nd edn.
● Green (1983). *Basic Clinical Physiology*, pages 133–136.

## SOCIOLOGICAL FACTORS AFFECTING ELIMINATION

Elimination is affected by the environment we live in and by the habits and practices of individuals in society. As far as environmental factors are concerned different communities and societies make various provisions for the safe and acceptable disposal of human waste, such as in modern sewage disposal plants sited on the outskirts of a city or town, in chemical closets for small isolated houses or caravans, or septic tanks in rural settings. Cultural background can influence individuals eliminating, by their choice of diet, fluid intake, habit training of their young, position adopted when micturating and defaecating, hygiene practices and need for privacy.

The main risks to the individuals from inadequate disposal of excreta are from faecal contamination of the water supply and transmission of intestinal pathogenic organisms by the faecal-oral route. Health Education and advice to travellers and holidaymakers helps to reduce the vulnerability of individuals who can also be protected by vaccination and immunisation, e.g. *Salmonella typhi* and *Salmonella paratyphi* A and B (TAB).

If we measure the vulnerability of the individual on a scale 1–10 and the adequacy of the disposal of human excreta as a scale 1–10, with 1 being the safest and 10 being the least safe, we can use the following chart (*Figure 5.1*) to illustrate how the adequacy of disposal of human excreta and the vulnerability of the individual are closely related.

**Figure 5.1** *Chart to illustrate the interrelationship of safe disposal of human excreta and the vulnerability of the individual*

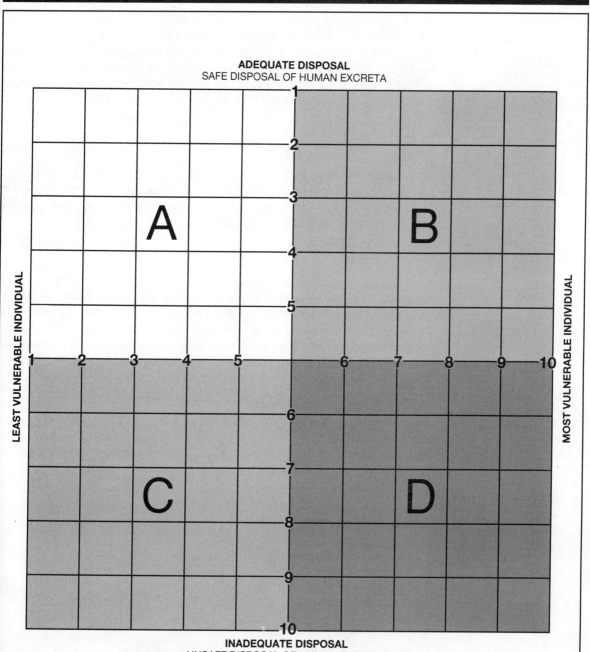

### Interrelationship of Adequate, Safe Disposal of Human Excreta and the Vulnerability of the Individual

We would like you to use the chart (*Figure 5.2*) as a graph by inserting a cross using the two scales from the following examples.

*Mrs Harding* lives in a city suburb in a modern housing development with her husband and two children. The house has a water closet (WC) and is connected to the city main drainage and sewage system. Mrs Harding ensures that her children wash their hands after eliminating and before eating. The family travel abroad regularly and they are fully protected by vaccination against enteric diseases.

Scale 1   Vulnerability
Scale 1   Adequacy of disposal

*Mr Smith* is helping to look after his teenage son who has developed diarrhoea on return from a camping holiday. They live in a recently renovated dwelling in an inner city area. Later he finds he has developed similar symptoms, having failed to observe adequate hand washing during his son's illness.

Scale 8   Vulnerability
Scale 2   Adequacy of disposal

*Mr Livingstone* prepared for his trip to the tropics by ensuring that he was fully vaccinated against enteric diseases as recommended by the travel agent, including TAB, anti-cholera and polio. He finds on arrival that the conditions available for eliminating are grossly inadequate and disposal of excreta is unsafe. Despite all possible precautions he develops diarrhoea and abdominal pain which is later found to be due to a virulent *Entamoeba coli*.

Scale 2    Vulnerability
Scale 10   Adequacy of disposal

*The Brown family* go on a caravan holiday in the Mediterranean. They have never been abroad before and have not sought any advice regarding protection against enteric diseases, nor have they provided an adequate disposal unit in the caravan.

Scale 10   Vulnerability
Scale 8    Adequacy of disposal

**Figure 5.2**   *Completed chart to illustrate the interrelationship of the safe disposal of human excreta and vulnerability of the individual*

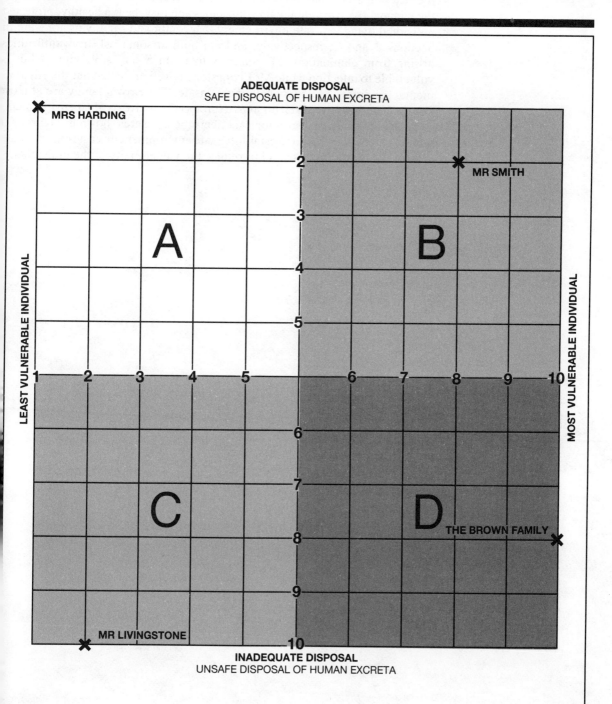

From the completed chart, *Figure 5.2*, you can now see into which sections the different individuals fit. Mrs Harding is in Section A: this section illustrates the minimal risk from eliminating difficulties and that she is a healthy, protected individual living in a safe environment. Mr Smith and Mr Livingstone are in Sections B and C, respectively, and are both at some risk from difficulties arising from elimination. Mr Smith is living in a safe environment but is vulnerable to infection while Mr Livingstone is well protected but the environmental conditions are overwhelmingly unsafe. The Brown family are at most risk because they have taken no steps to protect themselves or their environment.

To minimise adverse sociological effects the measures shown in *Figures 5.3* and *5.4* can be considered to establish a safe environment by ensuring adequate disposal of human excreta and to reduce the vulnerability of the individual.

**Figure 5.3**   *Factors which help to ensure safe disposal of human excreta*

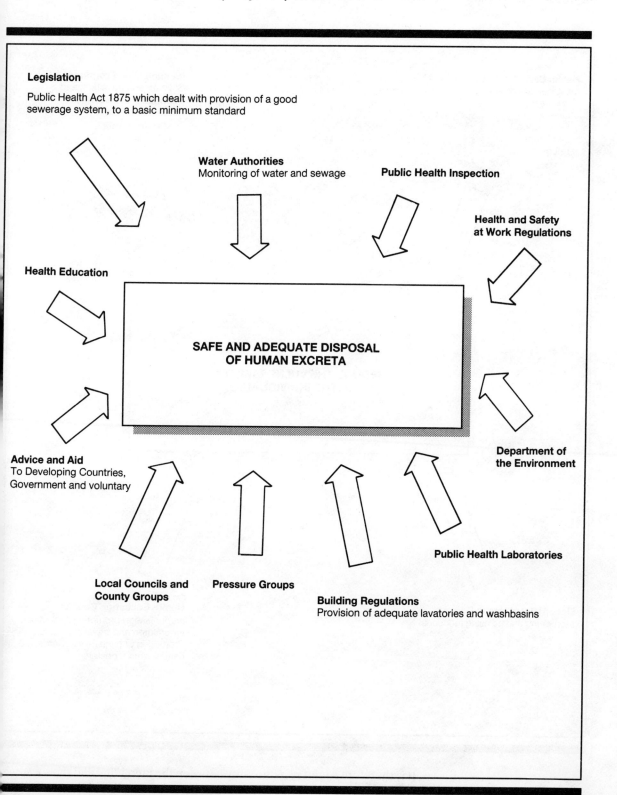

**Figure 5.4**   *Factors which help to reduce the vulnerability of the individual*

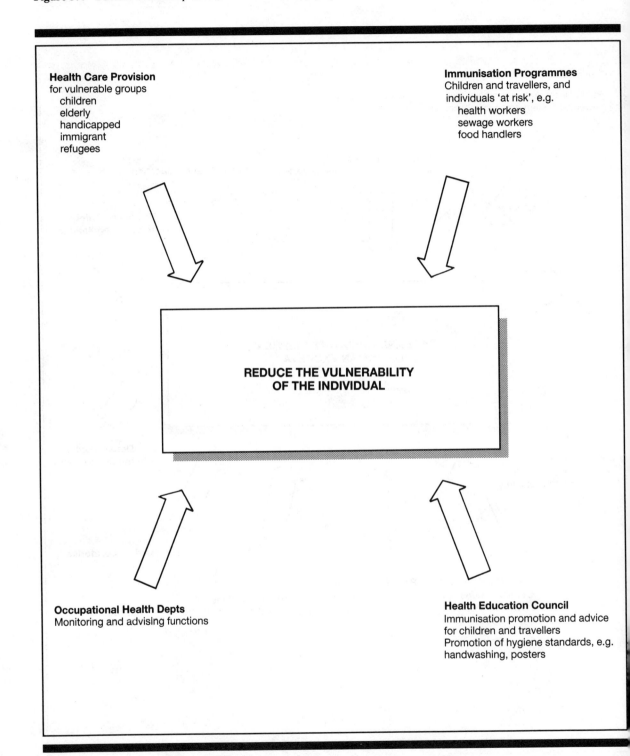

It is therefore a joint responsibility between the individual and the society he lives in to reduce risk and provide protection.

## PSYCHOLOGICAL FACTORS AFFECTING ELIMINATION

**Figure 5.5**  *Some psychological factors affecting elimination*

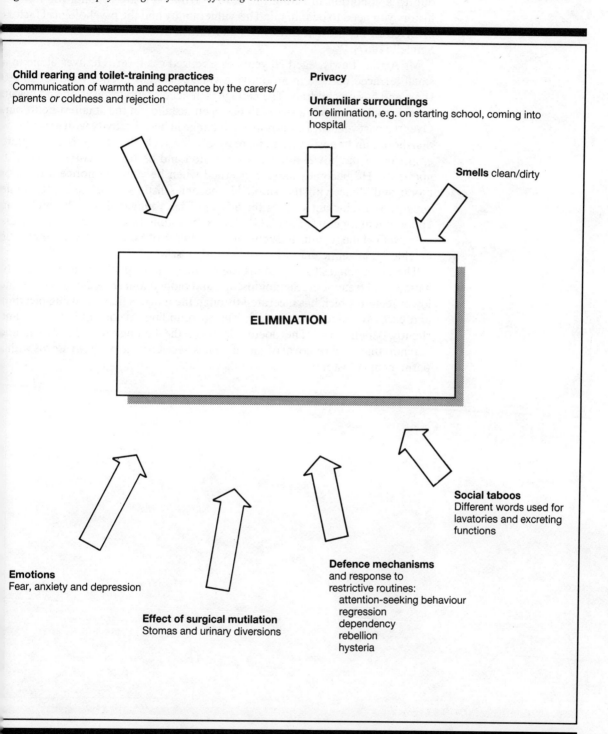

For further information see Boore (1980) and Tierney (1980).

### PATIENT HISTORY

We would now like you to consider a patient who has difficulty in eliminating due to a condition affecting the bowel. While you are reading Mr Lewis's history you need to bear in mind his vulnerability and the psychological factors involved in his present difficulties and future treatment. See also Hunt and Sendell (1987).

Mr Arthur Lewis, aged 70 years, is a retired gas fitter. He lives alone in a small terraced cottage in an outlying village. He has been a widower for 10 years and has no children. The cottage is in need of modernisation and has an outside toilet only but a sitz bath has been installed in the smallest bedroom. Over the past year Mr Lewis noticed a change in bowel activity with episodes of diarrhorea and constipation. Increasingly, he feels that there is incomplete emptying of the bowel after a bowel action and he tries to correct this with aperients. He becomes more concerned when he starts to notice a trace of blood and slime with the stool. He becomes listless, pale and loses some weight, and reluctantly takes the advice of his younger sister who makes an appointment for him to see his GP. On examination the doctor discovers a mass in the wall of the rectum and general examination of Mr Lewis reveals him to be an elderly, anaemic man who has recently lost weight.

The GP arranges for his admission to the local hospital for further investigations and treatment. Sigmoidoscopy and biopsy confirm a carcinoma of the lower rectum which has ulcerated through the mucous lining causing bleeding and excessive mucous secretion. The surrounding mucous lining is red and slightly oedematous. The doctor discusses the findings with Mr Lewis and explains that total removal of the rectum is necessary, leaving Mr Lewis with a permanent colostomy.

## EXPLANATION OF CLINICAL FEATURES

The clinical features of the disease affecting Mr Lewis's lower bowel are explained in *Table 5.1*.

*Table 5.1  Explanation of clinical features*

| Normal physiology | Abnormal physiology | Clinical features |
|---|---|---|
| The large intestine receives undigested food residues, e.g. cellulose, some insoluble compounds, bacteria, intestinal cells, mucus, cholesterol and bile pigments, and water from the small intestine | The large intestine continues to receive residue as normal. Even if the patient does not eat much, bacteria, intestinal cells, mucus, cholesterol and bile pigments and water still come from the small intestine and faeces are produced | None |
| By peristaltic action the residue is moved on towards the rectum. During this passage, water is reabsorbed into the bloodstream and the mucous lining produces mucus to lubricate the passageway. The faeces 'queue up' in the descending and sigmoid colon and are eliminated via the rectum and anus | A carcinoma growing in the lower rectum will cause an obstruction to the lumen of the bowel. The lumen becomes narrower as the carcinoma grows, so the passage of faeces becomes more difficult. Peristalsis increases initially. The residue builds up in the sigmoid colon proximal to the obstruction and the longer it is held up the more water is re-absorbed into the bloodstream | Colicky, lower abdominal pain Constipation and difficulty with defaecation Feeling of incomplete emptying of the bowel after defaecation |
|  | As more and more constipated faeces accumulate in the colon, the watery residue still arriving from the small intestine tracks down between the hard faeces and the wall of the colon | Bouts of diarrhoea/constipation and sometimes faecal incontinence |
| The mucous lining of the large intestine and rectum is smooth, pink and moist | A carcinoma invading the lining of the rectum can ulcerate and cause bleeding and excessive mucus secretion | Blood and mucus (slime) in the stool Anaemia Listlessness |
| The alimentary system enables the ingestion, digestion, absorption, and utilisation of water and nutrients | Presence of a malignant tumour anywhere in the body can alter metabolic processes | Cachexia, listlessness and loss of weight |

## EFFECTS OF DIFFICULTY WITH ELIMINATING (DEFAECATING) ON OTHER LIVING ACTIVITIES

Elimination is normally carried out without distress, discomfort or embarrassment and ensures the periodic evacuation of waste products from the body in a way that is socially acceptable to the individual's cultural environment. If a person has difficulty in eliminating, the other living activities could be affected and this may alter the way in which his physiological, security, achievement and self-fulfilment needs are met.

**Difficulty with Eliminating (defaecation)**

1. *Breathing*
   Not affected.

2. *Eating and Drinking*
   Appetite depressed. Loss of interest in eating and perhaps fear of eating and worsening the effects of symptoms.

3. *Eliminating*
   Altered bowel habits, nature and frequency of defaecation.

4. *Sleeping and Resting*
   Could be disturbed due to diarrhoea, abdominal pain and distension, anxiety about changes in bowel function.

5. *Moving*
   Could be affected by lack of energy due to disease, loss of nutrients from diarrhoea and lack of nutrients due to poor dietary intake.

6. *Maintaining Body Temperature*
   Not affected.

7. *Keeping Body Clean*
   May require assistance due to lack of energy from insufficient nutrients. Need for more attention to hygiene following diarrhoea.

8. *Dressing Suitably*
   May require modification of clothing particularly if very young or elderly.

9. *Avoiding Dangers and Injuries*
   Risks of faecal-oral route contamination increased.

10. *Communicating*
    Difficulties may be experienced in talking about eliminating when it is a socially taboo subject. Therefore may be reluctant to seek medical advice.

11. *Worshipping*
    May not be able to worship in formal gatherings.

12. *Working*
    May be unable to follow normal work.

13. *Participating in Recreation*
    Dependent on physical capability and degree of incapacity.

14. *Learning to Satisfy Curiosity*
    May need re-educating about bowel activity and how to cope with presenting problems.

## A METHOD TO ASSIST YOU IN ASSESSING MR LEWIS

As before we would now like you to complete the top half of the assessment sheet (*Figure 5.6*) and then proceed to use the information to decide which of Mr Lewis's total needs (physiological, security, achievement and self fulfilment) may be altered for him as an individual at this time. As a guide refer to the sample profiles in Section 1, Chapter 2, numbers 9 and 14 and decide how Mr Lewis is different. Check your ideas with the complete profile shown in *Figure 5.7*.

**Figure 5.6** *A patient profile to assist in assessing patients and the development of a problem-solving approach to care*

---

Name ___Mr Lewis_____ No. _____

Address _____

_____

Circle any features that are present in your patient in each of the five columns. Remember that more than one is possible in most of the columns

Section A  1. Starting with the age column, take your selected condition and consider each of the 14 functions requiring assistance and tick in the box(es) those appropriate to your patient's needs, e.g. an elderly patient may require assistance with 2, 3 and 5

Section B  2. Repeat the same procedure with subsequent columns

**(A) Conditions always present that affect basic needs**　　　　　　**Physiological disturbances**

| *Age* | *Temperament* | *Social/Cultural* | *Physical/Intellectual Capacity* | |
|---|---|---|---|---|
| Newborn | Emotional state | Member of a family | Normal weight | 1. Fluid and electrolyte imbalance |
| Child | or passing mode: | unit with friends | Over-weight | 2. Oxygen want |
| Adolescent | (a) normal | and status | Under-weight | 3. Shock |
| Adult | (b) euphoric, | A person relatively | Normal mentality | 4. Consciousness |
| Middle aged | hyperactive | alone | Gifted mentality | 5. Local injury/ disease |
| Elderly | (c) anxious, fearful, | Maladjusted | Normal sense of: | 6. Metabolism |
| Aged | agitated, | Destitute | hearing | 7. Seeing, hearing, smell and touch |
| | hysterical | Smoker | sight | 8. Communicable conditions |
| | (d) depressed/ | Drinker | equilibrium | 9. Immobilisation: disease/treatment |
| | hypoactive | | touch | |
| | | | Loss of sense of: | |
| | | | hearing | |
| | | | sight | |
| | | | equilibrium | |
| | | | touch | |
| | | | Normal motor power | |
| | | | Loss of motor power | |

**(B)**

| Functions requiring assistance | Age | Temperament | Social/Cultural | Physical/Intellectual Capacity | Physiological Disturbance |
|---|---|---|---|---|---|
| 1. Breathing | | | | | |
| 2. Eating or drinking | | | | | |
| 3. Elimination | | | | | |
| 4. Sleep or rest | | | | | |
| 5. Movement | | | | | |
| 6. Maintenance of body temperature | | | | | |
| 7. Keeping body clean | | | | | |
| 8. Dressing suitably | | | | | |
| 9. Avoiding dangers and injury | | | | | |
| 10. Communication | | | | | |
| 11. Worship | | | | | |
| 12. Work | | | | | |
| 13. Participation in recreation | | | | | |
| 14. Learning to satisfy curiosity | | | | | |

**Figure 5.7** *Profile for Mr Lewis before admission to hospital*

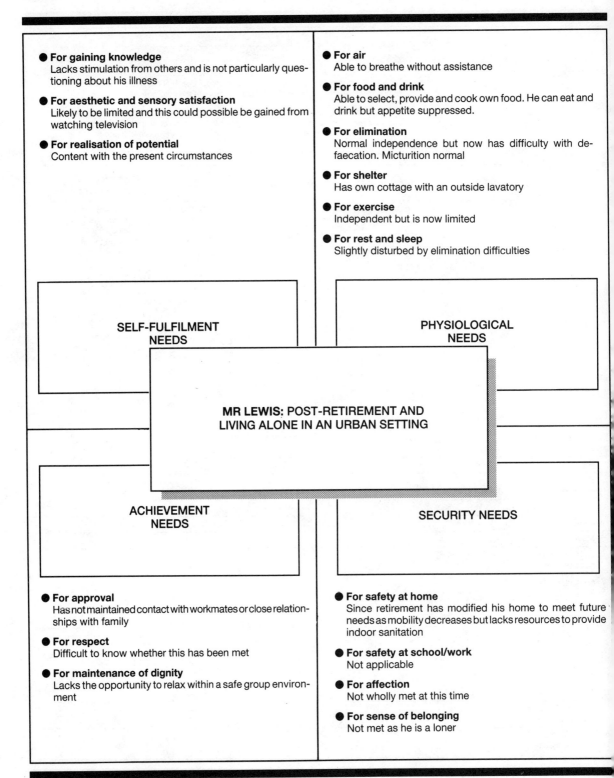

● **For gaining knowledge**
Lacks stimulation from others and is not particularly questioning about his illness

● **For aesthetic and sensory satisfaction**
Likely to be limited and this could possible be gained from watching television

● **For realisation of potential**
Content with the present circumstances

● **For air**
Able to breathe without assistance

● **For food and drink**
Able to select, provide and cook own food. He can eat and drink but appetite suppressed.

● **For elimination**
Normal independence but now has difficulty with defaecation. Micturition normal

● **For shelter**
Has own cottage with an outside lavatory

● **For exercise**
Independent but is now limited

● **For rest and sleep**
Slightly disturbed by elimination difficulties

SELF-FULFILMENT
NEEDS

PHYSIOLOGICAL
NEEDS

MR LEWIS: POST-RETIREMENT AND
LIVING ALONE IN AN URBAN SETTING

ACHIEVEMENT
NEEDS

SECURITY NEEDS

● **For approval**
Has not maintained contact with workmates or close relationships with family

● **For respect**
Difficult to know whether this has been met

● **For maintenance of dignity**
Lacks the opportunity to relax within a safe group environment

● **For safety at home**
Since retirement has modified his home to meet future needs as mobility decreases but lacks resources to provide indoor sanitation

● **For safety at school/work**
Not applicable

● **For affection**
Not wholly met at this time

● **For sense of belonging**
Not met as he is a loner

You are now in a position to complete the lower section of the Assessment Sheet (*Figure 5.6*). Starting with the age column take your selected feature previously circled and consider each of the fourteen functions requiring assistance and tick in the boxes those appropriate to Mr Lewis's needs. Repeat the same procedure with the subsequent columns. Check your completed Assessment Sheet with the one that follows, *Figure 5.8*.

**Figure 5.8** *A patient profile to assist in assessing patients and the development of a problem-solving approach to care*

Name _____ Mr Lewis _____ No. _____

Address _____

Circle any features that are present in your patient in each of the five columns. Remember that more than one is possible in most of the columns

Section A 1. Starting with the age column, take your selected condition and consider each of the 14 functions requiring assistance and tick in the box(es) those appropriate to your patient's needs, e.g. an elderly patient may require assistance with 2, 3 and 5

Section B 2. Repeat the same procedure with subsequent columns

**(A) Conditions always present that affect basic needs**

**Physiological disturbances**

| *Age* | *Temperament* | *Social/Cultural* | *Physical/Intellectual Capacity* | |
|---|---|---|---|---|
| Newborn | Emotional state | Member of a family | | 1. Fluid and electrolyte imbalance |
| Child | or passing mode: | unit with friends and status | Normal weight | 2. Oxygen want |
| Adolescent | (a) normal | A person relatively | Over-weight | 3. Shock |
| Adult | (b) euphoric, hyperactive | alone | Under-weight | 4. Consciousness |
| Middle aged | | Maladjusted | Normal mentality | 5. Local injury/disease |
| Elderly | (c) anxious, fearful, agitated, hysterical | Destitute | Gifted mentality | 6. Metabolism |
| Aged | | Smoker | Normal sense of: | 7. Seeing, hearing, smell and touch |
| | (d) depressed/hypoactive | Drinker | hearing | 8. Communicable conditions |
| | | | sight | 9. Immobilisation: disease/treatment |
| | | | equilibrium | |
| | | | touch | |
| | | | Loss of sense of: | |
| | | | hearing | |
| | | | sight | |
| | | | equilibrium | |
| | | | touch | |
| | | | Normal motor power | |
| | | | Loss of motor power | |

**(B)**

| Functions requiring assistance | *Age* | *Temperament* | *Social/Cultural* | *Physical/Intellectual Capacity* | *Physiological Disturbance* |
|---|---|---|---|---|---|
| 1. Breathing | | | | | |
| 2. Eating or drinking | | | | | ✓ |
| 3. Elimination | | | | | ✓ |
| 4. Sleep or rest | | | | | ✓ |
| 5. Movement | | | | | ✓ |
| 6. Maintenance of body temperature | | | | | |
| 7. Keeping body clean | | | | | ✓ |
| 8. Dressing suitably | | | | | ? Possible |
| 9. Avoiding dangers and injury | | | | | ✓ |
| 10. Communication | | | ✓ | | ✓ |
| 11. Worship | | | | | |
| 12. Work | | | | | |
| 13. Participation in recreation | | | | | ✓ |
| 14. Learning to satisfy curiosity | | | ✓ | | ✓ |

You now know that Mr Lewis's social setting and disease process has a particular effect on his ability to meet his physiological, security, achievement and self-fulfilment needs.

## SELECTING NURSING ACTIONS TO ASSIST A PATIENT WITH DIFFICULTY IN ELIMINATING

The main problem being discussed in this chapter is *difficulty in eliminating* and in this part a patient with difficulty in *defaecation*. We would now like you to choose from the list of nursing actions shown in *Table 5.2* those appropriate for Mr Lewis by putting a tick in either the Yes column if you think the action is appropriate, in the No column if you think the action is inappropriate or dangerous or in the Maybe column if you think the action is possible. Whatever your decision give an explanation for each of your choices and when you have completed this compare your decision and explanations with those given on pages 128–130.

Table 5.2   *Nursing action to assist a patient with difficulty in eliminating*

| Nursing actions | Yes | No | Maybe | Reason for choice |
|---|---|---|---|---|
| **Part 1   Breathing** | | | | |
| 1. Provide extra pillows at night | | | | |
| **Part 2   Eating and Drinking** | | | | |
| 1. Offer a normal diet | | | | |
| 2. Offer a high fibre diet | | | | |
| 3. Offer a low residue diet | | | | |
| 4. Offer a fluid diet | | | | |
| 5. Offer a high protein diet | | | | |
| 6. Encourage patient to drink hourly | | | | |
| 7. Advise patient to restrict amount of fluid drunk | | | | |
| 8. Discover likes and dislikes | | | | |
| 9. Assist in completing menu requests | | | | |
| **Part 3   Eliminating** | | | | |
| 1. Give suppositories | | | | |
| 2. Give an enema | | | | |
| 3. Give an aperient | | | | |
| 4. Allow patient to go to toilet as required using a bedpan or urinal | | | | |

*Table 5.2    Continued*

| Nursing actions | Yes | No | Maybe | Reason for choice |
|---|---|---|---|---|
| **Part 3    Eliminating (continued)** | | | | |
| 5. Offer bedpan as required | | | | |
| 6. Offer commode day or night | | | | |
| 7. Perform manual evacuation | | | | |
| 8. Give rectal/colon washouts | | | | |
| 9. Prepare patient for sigmoidoscopy, biopsy and/ or barium enema | | | | |
| **Part 4    Sleeping and Resting** | | | | |
| 1. Offer warm drink at night | | | | |
| 2. Ensure adequate ventilation in the ward | | | | |
| 3. Position patient's bed near the toilet | | | | |
| 4. Position patient's bed at top-end of ward away from toilets | | | | |
| 5. Offer night sedation | | | | |
| **Part 5    Moving** | | | | |
| 1. Keep patient at complete rest | | | | |
| 2. Encourage exercise | | | | |
| 3. Sit in easy chair | | | | |
| 4. Assist in repositioning in bed | | | | |
| 5. Provide a sheepskin | | | | |
| 6. Provide a ripple bed | | | | |
| 7. Provide a hoist | | | | |
| **Part 6    Maintaining Body Temperature** | | | | |
| 1. Provide plenty of blankets | | | | |
| 2. Provide light bed clothes | | | | |
| **Part 7    Keeping Body Clean** | | | | |
| 1. Give daily bed bath | | | | |
| 2. Assist patient washing in bed | | | | |

*Table 5.2   Continued*

| Nursing actions | Yes | No | Maybe | Reason for choice |
|---|---|---|---|---|
| **Part 7   Keeping Body Clean (continued)** | | | | |
| 3. Assist patient washing in bathroom | | | | |
| 4. Encourage patient to bath | | | | |
| 5. Assist patient to shave and brush hair | | | | |
| 6. Provide opportunity to wash after eliminating | | | | |
| 7. Offer antiseptic mouthwashes | | | | |
| 8. Give oral toilet | | | | |
| **Part 8   Dressing Suitably** | | | | |
| 1. Provide hospital pyjamas | | | | |
| 2. Provide hospital dressing gown and slippers | | | | |
| 3. Encourage use of own pyjamas | | | | |
| 4. Encourage to be up and dressed during the day | | | | |
| 5. Provide aids to prevent soiling of clothing | | | | |
| **Part 9   Avoiding Dangers and Injury** | | | | |
| 1. Provide facilities for adequate hand washing after eliminating | | | | |
| **Part 10   Communicating** | | | | |
| 1. Allocate a nurse to the patient | | | | |
| 2. Assist in contact with relatives | | | | |
| 3. Give an opportunity for exchange of information with patient, relatives and staff | | | | |
| 4. Encourage him to participate in conversation with staff | | | | |
| 5. Position patient's bed in the middle of the ward to promote social interaction | | | | |
| 6. Position patient's bed in a side ward to provide privacy | | | | |
| 7. Make an appointment for stoma therapist to visit | | | | |
| **Part 11   Worshipping** | | | | |
| 1. Inform hospital chaplain | | | | |

*Table 5.2　Continued*

| Nursing actions | Yes | No | Maybe | Reason for choice |
|---|---|---|---|---|
| **Part 11　Worshipping (continued)**<br><br>2. Inform patient's own chaplain of patient's admission<br><br>3. Ignore spiritual needs until patient is feeling better | | | | |
| **Part 12　Working**<br><br>　Not appropriate as patient is retired and not in permanent employment | | | | |
| **Part 13　Participating in Recreation**<br><br>1. Provide formal occupational therapy<br><br>2. Assist patient in using the television room | | | | |
| **Part 14　Learning to Satisfy Curiosity**<br><br>1. Keep patient fully informed of condition and progress<br><br>2. Avoid discussing problems of elimination | | | | |

## EXPLANATION FOR CHOICE OF NURSING ACTIONS

### *Part 1　Breathing*

You should have ticked the Yes column remembering that Mr Lewis is anaemic and the oxygen carrying capacity of his blood is reduced. He may breathe more easily sitting up to allow full expansion of his lungs.

### *Part 2　Eating and Drinking*

We hope you have ticked the Yes column for numbers 3, 8 and 9. A low residue diet will help to minimise the amount of faecal material produced to overcome the obstruction in the lower bowel. Mr Lewis will need assistance in choosing an appropriate diet when completing his menu and as far as possible his likes and dislikes will need to be taken into account. You should have ticked the Maybe column for numbers 3, 4 and 5. A fluid diet may be ordered prior to investigation and/or surgery, or to minimise the risk of acute intestinal obstruction. A high protein diet may be appropriate if Mr Lewis's nutritional state is poor and constipation may be helped if he is encouraged to increase his fluid intake. You should have ticked numbers 2 and 7 in the No column. A normal or high fibre diet would be inappropriate for Mr Lewis as it would increase the bulk of the faecal residue and increase the risk of obstruction. Restricting the amount of fluid drunk increases the reabsorption of fluid from the gut in the body's effort to maintain fluid hydration, so this could exacerbate constipation.

## Part 3   Eliminating

We hope you have ticked the Yes column for numbers 2, 4, 5, 8 and 9. Mr Lewis will be given an enema and rectal/colon washout to prepare the bowel for sigmoidoscopy biopsy and/or barium enema and eventually surgery. Numbers 4 and 5 need to be offered as his condition requires. You should have ticked the Maybe column for numbers 1, 6 and 7. Suppositories may be used to empty the lower rectum distal to the obstruction. If faecal impaction has occurred manual evacuation may be necessary. Number 6 depends on his mobility, general condition and preference. Number 3 should be in the No column since an aperient would cause unnecessary abdominal pain and possibly perforation of the gut.

## Part 4   Sleeping and Resting

Numbers 1, 2 and 3 should be in the Yes column. Numbers 1 and 2 can assist in settling and providing comfort to the patient while number 3 should enable the patient to get to the toilet without having far to go and having to disturb other patients. Number 4 should be ticked in the No column for the opposite reason to number 3. Number 5, night sedation, could be helpful in assisting Mr Lewis to get adequate sleep and rest.

## Part 5   Moving

We hope you have ticked numbers 2 and 3 in the Yes column as it is important to maintain his present mobility and independence. If he is weak then you should have ticked the Maybe column for numbers 4, 5 and 7; by helping him to reposition himself in bed and with the use of a sheepskin and hoist you would assist in preventing the risks of bedrest. The No column should be ticked for numbers 1 and 6 as neither are appropriate for Mr Lewis at the time.

## Part 6   Maintaining Body Temperature

Mr Lewis may require extra or less bedclothes depending on his personal preference, but may have a tendency to feel cold due to his recent loss of weight and anaemia.

## Part 7   Keeping the Body Clean

We hope you have ticked the Yes column for numbers 4, 5, 6 and 7. Encouraging the patient to bath himself and assisting him to shave and brush his hair maintains some independence. Perianal skin may become excoriated unless meticulous hygiene is used following eliminating, especially during bouts of diarrhoea. There is a risk of oral infection if the patient's appetite is suppressed and he is not enjoying a normal diet. You should have ticked numbers 2, 3 and 8 in the Maybe column: these nursing actions may be appropriate if Mr Lewis is more dependent. You should have ticked the No column for number 1 as it is unlikely that Mr Lewis is this dependent.

## Part 8   Dressing Suitably

You should have ticked the Yes column for numbers 3, 4 and 5 as using his own clothes and getting up and dressed during the day helps Mr Lewis to maintain his independence and dignity. Number 5 needs to be considered if the patient has urgency, leakage or incontinence: modifications of clothing

may be needed to assist in quicker and easy removal. You should have
ticked numbers 1 and 2 in the Maybe column, remembering that Mr Lewis
lives alone and may have difficulty in obtaining freshly laundered clothes.

### Part 9   Avoiding Dangers and Injury

You should have ticked the Yes column here. There is the danger of faecal-
oral contamination.

### Part 10   Communicating

You should have ticked the Yes column for numbers 1, 2, 3 and 4: all of
these are necessary as Mr Lewis has been socially isolated since his wife's
death and his retirement. You should also tick number 7 in the Yes column
to give opportunity for the stoma therapist to teach suitable after care and
use of appliances. For the same reason you could have ticked the Maybe
column for numbers 5 and 6, although these would depend on his wishes
and the facilities available.

### Part 11   Worshipping

Items 1 and 2 could have been ticked in the Maybe column depending on
the patient's wishes. Number 3 should be ticked in the No column. If
acknowledged by the patient, spiritual needs should be met promptly.

### Part 12   Working

As Mr Lewis is retired this section is not appropriate.

### Part 13   Participating in Recreation

You could have ticked number 2 in the Yes column as it is likely that this
form of entertainment is used by him normally. Number 1 should be ticked
in the No column as formal occupational therapy is not appropriate for Mr
Lewis at this time.

### Part 14   Learning to Satisfy Curiosity

You should have ticked Yes for number 1 as Mr Lewis should be kept
informed even though he may not appear to be questioning about his condition. Item 2 should have been ticked in the No column: he has difficulty
with elimination and should be encouraged to verbalise his fears and anxieties
on what could be a difficult subject.

## CHOOSING PRIORITIES IN NURSING ACTIONS

It can be seen that some of these nursing actions are dependent on the
individual characteristics of Mr Lewis and therefore his care plan needs to
be sensitive to his individual needs. As we have suggested before you may
like to discuss some of the answers we have suggested with your colleagues
and/or tutor, as this will help you to develop a questioning approach. Using
Table 5.3 identify your priorities for planning the care that Mr Lewis requires.

*Table 5.3   Priorities in nursing actions*

| Part | Insert your choice of priority numbers 1–14 |
|---|---|
| 1.  Breathing | |
| 2.  Eating and drinking | |
| 3.  Eliminating | |
| 4.  Sleeping and resting | |
| 5.  Moving | |
| 6.  Maintaining body temperature | |
| 7.  Keeping body clean | |
| 8.  Dressing suitably | |
| 9.  Avoiding dangers and injury | |
| 10. Communicating | |
| 11. Worshipping | |
| 12. Working | |
| 13. Participating in recreation | |
| 14. Learning to satisfy curiosity | |

You can now check your decision regarding priority choice of Nursing Actions with the plan in *Table 5.4*. As you can see Part 3 is our first priority for Mr Lewis. If you wish to remind yourself about planning and providing nursing care refer again to *Table 3.4*.

## IDENTIFICATION OF CRITERIA OF PROGRESS

You should now read carefully the plan shown in *Table 5.4* which identifies criteria for progress.

*Table 5.4   Plan of care for progress*

| Nursing actions to assist a patient with difficulty in defaecating | Yes | Maybe | Priority Choice | Measurements | Short-term goals | Review period | Evaluation Criteria Have short-term goals been met? |
|---|---|---|---|---|---|---|---|
| **Part 3   Eliminating**<br>1. Give suppositories<br>2. Give an enema<br>4. Allow patient to go to toilet as required using a bedpan or urinal<br>5. Offer bedpan as required<br>6. Offer commode day or night<br>7. Perform manual evacuation<br>8. Give rectal/colon washouts<br>9. Prepare patient for sigmoidoscopy biopsy and/or barium enema | ✓ (2)<br>✓ (4)<br>✓ (5)<br>✓ (8)<br>✓ (9) | ✓ (1)<br>✓ (6)<br>✓ (7) | FIRST | Record:<br>(a) Frequency, consistency, amount of bowel actions<br>(b) Presence of blood or mucus<br>(c) Passage of flatus<br>(d) Presence of discomfort and abdominal/rectal pain<br>(e) Incontinence, leakage | Prevent accumulation of faecal matter distal and proximal to obstruction<br><br>To prepare the bowel for examination and surgery | Twice daily | The first two rectal washouts produced a return of fair amount of faecal matter. Washings now clear. Passing flatus. Abdomen soft, not distended. Patient still has sensation of incomplete emptying of rectum and some abdominal pain |
| **Part 2   Eating and Drinking**<br>3. Offer a low residue diet<br>4. Offer a fluid diet<br>5. Offer a high protein diet<br>6. Encourage patient to drink hourly<br>8. Discover likes and dislikes<br>9. Assist in completing menu requests | ✓ (3)<br>✓ (8)<br>✓ (9) | ✓ (4)<br>✓ (5)<br>✓ (6) | SECOND | Record:<br>(a) How much food and fluid is eaten and drunk<br>(b) Frequency of taking food and drink<br>(c) When he feels hungry<br>(d) Type of intake, likes and dislikes<br>(e) Weight | (a), (b), (c), (d) Intake of 2 litres of fluid and 2000 calories in 24 hours and not feeling hungry<br><br><br>(e) Provide a base line for surgery | (a), (b), (c), (d)<br>24-hourly<br><br><br>(e) Prior to discharge | Drinking 2 litres of fluid but consumed 1000 calories only<br><br>Missing his usual foods and has little interest in meals<br><br>Weight 60 kg |
| **Part 4   Sleeping and Resting**<br>1. Offer warm drink at night<br>2. Ensure adequate ventilation in the ward | ✓ (1)<br>✓ (2) | | THIRD | Record:<br>(a) Length of sleep<br>(b) Number of times up to toilet at night<br>(c) Whether night sedation required | 6–7 hours undisturbed sleep or rest | 24-hourly (a.m.) | Disturbed 4 times during the first night due to need to eliminate<br><br>Tired on rising |

*Table 5.4   Continued*

| Nursing actions to assist a patient with difficulty in defaecating | Yes | Maybe | Priority Choice | Measurements | Short-term goals | Review period | Evaluation Criteria Have short-term goals been met? |
|---|---|---|---|---|---|---|---|
| **Part 4 Sleeping and Resting (continued)** | | | | | | | |
| 3. Position patient's bed near the toilet | ✓ | | | | | | |
| 5. Offer night sedation | | ✓ | THIRD | | | | |
| **Part 1   Breathing** | | | | | | | |
| 1. Provide extra pillows at night | ✓ | | | | | | |
| **Part 10 Communicating** | | | FOURTH | Note levels of anxiety/frustration from patient and relative | Mr Lewis is content with care being given and feels able to relate to staff | Ongoing | Mr Lewis's sister is visiting daily. Medical staff have discussed progress and prognosis with both Mr Lewis and his sister |
| 1. Allocate a nurse to the patient | ✓ | | | | | | |
| 2. Assist in contact with relatives | ✓ | | | | | | Mr Lewis has asked not to have the chaplain informed |
| 3. Give an opportunity for exchange of information with patient, relatives and staff | ✓ | | | | | | Waiting for the stoma therapist to visit |
| 4. Encourage him to participate in conversation with staff | ✓ | | | | | | |
| 5. Position patient's bed in the middle of the ward to promote social interaction | | ✓ | | | | | |
| 6. Position patient's bed in a side ward to provide privacy | | ✓ | | | | | |
| 7. Make an appointment for stoma therapist to visit | ✓ | | | | | | |
| **Part 11   Worshipping** | | | | | | | |
| 1. Inform hospital chaplain | | ✓ | | | | | |
| 2. Inform patient's own chaplain of patient's admission | | ✓ | | | | | |

*Table 5.4   Continued*

| Nursing actions to assist a patient with difficulty in defaecating. | Yes | Maybe | Priority Choice | Measurements | Short-term goals | Review period | Evaluation Criteria Have short-term goals been met? |
|---|---|---|---|---|---|---|---|
| **Part 14   Learning to Satisfy Curiosity**<br>1. Keep patient fully informed of condition and progress | ✓ | | FOURTH | | | | |
| **Part 9   Avoiding Dangers and Injury**<br>1. Provide facilities for adequate hand washing after eliminating | ✓ | | FIFTH | Note whether Mr Lewis is attentive to personal hygiene | Minimise risk of cross-infection | Ongoing | Mr Lewis is meticulous about his personal hygiene |
| **Part 5   Moving**<br>2. Encourage exercise | ✓ | | | Note Mr Lewis's level of activity | That Mr Lewis gets adequate rest to compensate for disturbances | 24-hourly | Spending most of the day resting on his bed. Walking to toilet as required |
| 3. Sit in easy chair | ✓ | | | | | | |
| 4. Assist in repositioning in bed | | ✓ | | | | | |
| 5. Provide a sheepskin | | ✓ | | | | | |
| 7. Provide a hoist | | ✓ | | | | | |
| **Part 6   Maintaining Body Temperature**<br>1. Provide plenty of blankets | | ✓ | SIXTH | Record body temperature daily | Body temperature remains within normal limits | 24-hourly | Body temperature within normal limits |
| 2. Provide light bedclothes | | ✓ | | | | | |
| **Part 8   Dressing Suitably**<br>1. Provide hospital pyjamas | | ✓ | | Note that Mr Lewis dresses daily in his own clothes<br><br>Check discreetly for any soiling of own clothes and offer aids | Minimise any loss of dignity and independence | 24-hourly | Mr Lewis uses his own clothes during the day and has been given a supply of small disposable pads |
| 2. Provide hospital dressing gown and slippers | | ✓ | | | | | |
| 3. Encourage use of own pyjamas | ✓ | | | | | | |
| 4. Encourage to be up and dressed during the day | ✓ | | | | | | |
| 5. Provide aids to prevent soiling of clothing | ✓ | | | | | | |

*Table 5.4 Continued*

| Nursing actions to assist a patient with difficulty in defaecating. | Yes | Maybe | Priority Choice | Measurements | Short-term goals | Review period | Evaluation Criteria Have short-term goals been met? |
|---|---|---|---|---|---|---|---|
| **Part 13 Participating in Recreation**<br><br>2. Assist patient in using the television room | ✓ | | SEVENTH | Note Mr Lewis's interest in outside affairs | Prevent boredom and brooding about present condition | Ongoing | Watches the news on television<br><br>Attention span short |

### Using Evaluation Criteria for Resetting Short-term Goals

From the previous chapters you know how to do this. We would like to suggest that you reconsider Mr Lewis's evaluation criteria at the end of the first 24 hours in hospital and decide on new priorities for nursing actions, revised measurements and setting new short-term goals for preparing him for surgical intervention (abdominoperineal excision of rectum).

## IDENTIFICATION OF LONG-TERM GOALS

We would expect that after surgery Mr Lewis would be able to return home, maintain his health and weight and care for the stoma under conditions as near normal as possible. He should be confident that professional help will be available as and when he requires it from the stoma therapist, GP and district nurse. If you use the individual profile of Mr Lewis before admission to hospital and the individual profiles numbers 9 and 14 in Chapter 2 you can complete a long-term goal profile which will indicate his expected level of independence for his age, social setting and physiological change in elmininating. Refer to *Figure 5.9.*

**Figure 5.9** *Long-term goal profile for Mr Lewis*

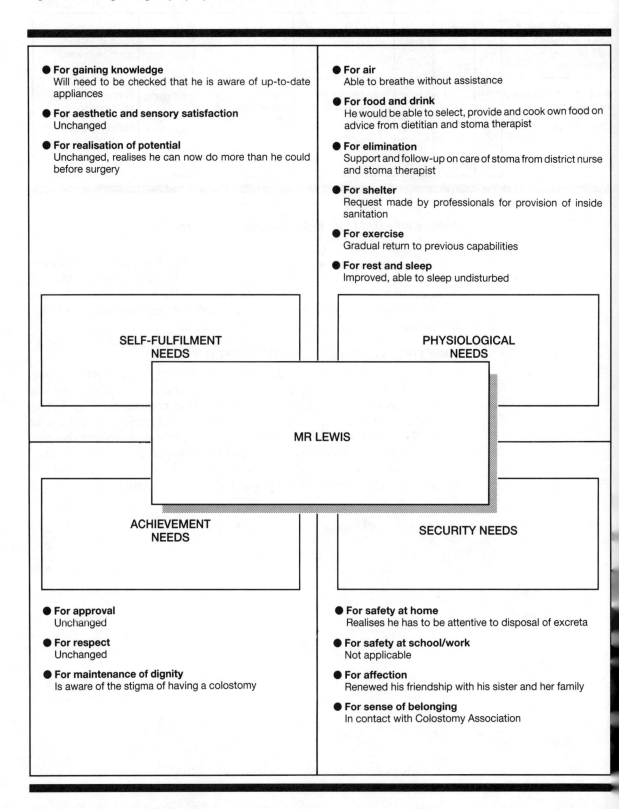

● **For gaining knowledge**
Will need to be checked that he is aware of up-to-date appliances

● **For aesthetic and sensory satisfaction**
Unchanged

● **For realisation of potential**
Unchanged, realises he can now do more than he could before surgery

● **For air**
Able to breathe without assistance

● **For food and drink**
He would be able to select, provide and cook own food on advice from dietitian and stoma therapist

● **For elimination**
Support and follow-up on care of stoma from district nurse and stoma therapist

● **For shelter**
Request made by professionals for provision of inside sanitation

● **For exercise**
Gradual return to previous capabilities

● **For rest and sleep**
Improved, able to sleep undisturbed

SELF-FULFILMENT
NEEDS

PHYSIOLOGICAL
NEEDS

MR LEWIS

ACHIEVEMENT
NEEDS

SECURITY NEEDS

● **For approval**
Unchanged

● **For respect**
Unchanged

● **For maintenance of dignity**
Is aware of the stigma of having a colostomy

● **For safety at home**
Realises he has to be attentive to disposal of excreta

● **For safety at school/work**
Not applicable

● **For affection**
Renewed his friendship with his sister and her family

● **For sense of belonging**
In contact with Colostomy Association

### Pharmacology and Suggested Nursing Procedures Related to Care of Patients with Difficulty in Defaecation

You may wish to familiarise yourself with medicine commonly used for patients with difficulty in *defaecation*:

Aperients
Bowel 'disinfectants'.

### Suggested Nursing Procedures / Guidelines for Nursing Practice

You may wish to familiarise yourself with your local policies and procedures/ guidelines for nursing practice which may be applicable to a patient requiring assistance with difficulty in *defaecation*.

Colonic lavage
Disposable enemas and suppositories
Radiological investigation
Colonoscopy
Sigmoidoscopy
Rectal examination

### PATIENT HISTORY

We would now like to consider a patient who has difficulty in eliminating due to a condition affecting micturition. While you are reading Mr Gibbard's history you need to bear in mind his vulnerability and psychological factors in his present difficulties. *Table 5.5* gives an explanation of the clinical features of the disease affecting Mr Gibbard's urinary system. See also Hunt and Sendell (1987).

Mr John Gibbard, aged 65 years, has recently retired from his job as a pharmacist. He has been looking forward to his retirement and forthcoming visit to America with his wife to visit their son and family. Six months before they were due to go to America he started to develop urinary symptoms: frequency of micturition during day and night, poor stream and difficulty in emptying his bladder completely. After a social evening with friends in the local pub he awoke during the night with a full bladder but was unable to pass urine. He became distressed and agitated and woke his wife. The doctor was contacted and he arranged for Mr Gibbard to be admitted to hospital.

On admission Mr Gibbard is found to be in severe pain with acute retention of urine, the bladder is distended and palpable above the symphysis pubis. Rectal examination reveals an enlarged prostate gland; Mr Gibbard is prepared for the insertion of a supra-pubic catheter and controlled decompression of the bladder. He is transferred to the surgical ward feeling much more comfortable and allowed to rest. The next morning the need for the following investigations are discussed:

1. Cystoscopy, biopsy of prostate gland and retrograde pyelogram.
2. Blood urea and electrolytes.
3. Haemoglobin and full blood count.
4. Specimen of urine for culture, sensitivity and microscopy.

Closed bladder drainage is continued and Mr Gibbard is encouraged to drink a minimum of three litres of fluid daily.

# EXPLANATION OF CLINICAL FEATURES

*Table 5.5 Abnormal physiology and clinical features*

| Normal physiology | Abnormal physiology | Clinical features |
|---|---|---|
| The bladder is a muscular bag which stores urine. The urethra is the passage which conveys urine from the bladder to the outside of the body | Continues to store urine normally | None |
| At the junction of the bladder and urethra is the internal sphincter. The prostate gland (in the male) surrounds the bladder neck<br><br>As the bladder fills the pressure within it rises and stimulates the desire to micturate | Prostate gland hypertrophies (enlarges) causing narrowing of the lumen of the urethra. Obstruction to the outflow of urine at the bladder neck causes the pressure to go on rising as the bladder continues to fill and distend | Bladder is palpable above the symphysis pubis<br><br>Abdominal pain<br><br>Rectal examination reveals palpable enlarged prostate gland |
| If convenient, micturition takes place:<br>   internal and external sphincters relax and open;<br>   the detrusor muscle in the bladder contracts the abdominal muscles and diaphragm contract and the bladder empties.<br><br>This normally occurs 3 to 4 times per day and rarely at night | Continues to attempt to empty the bladder through the obstruction<br><br>Incomplete emptying of the bladder | Frequency of micturition day and night. Feeling of incomplete emptying of the bladder despite increased effort of accessory muscles (abdominal). Urinary stream is weak in force and thin in calibre |
|  | Unusually large intake of fluid in a short space of time causes rapid over-distention of the bladder and pressure on the bladder outlet | Unable to pass any urine, increased pain, distressed. Bladder continues to distend further |

## EFFECTS OF DIFFICULTY WITH ELIMINATING (MICTURATING) ON OTHER LIVING ACTIVITIES

The effects of difficulty with micturating on other living activities are similar to those brought about by difficulty with defaecation. They may alter the way in which the patient's physiological, security, achievement and self-fulfilment needs are met.

### Difficulty with Eliminating (micturating)

1. *Breathing*
   Not affected.

2. *Eating and Drinking*
   Not affected until acute retention occurs.

3. *Eliminating*
   Altered micturition—bladder emptied more frequently, less efficiently.

4. *Sleeping and Resting*
   Disturbed day and night by frequency and difficulty in passing urine.

5. *Moving*
Restricted as access to lavatory is needed.

6. *Maintaining Body Temperature*
Not affected.

7. *Keeping Body Clean*
Not affected.

8. *Dressing Suitably*
Modification of clothing may be necessary particularly in the elderly.

9. *Avoiding Danger and Injury*
No particular risk.

10. *Communicating*
Difficulties may be experienced in talking about eliminating when it is a socially taboo subject. Therefore may be reluctant to question medical advice.

11. *Worshipping*
May not be able to worship in formal gatherings.

12. *Working*
May be unable to follow normal work.

13. *Participating in Recreation*
Dependent on physical capability and degree of incapacity.

14. *Learning to Satisfy Curiosity*
Needs information about the effects of surgery.

## ASSESSING MR GIBBARD

We would now like you to complete the top half of the assessment sheet shown in *Figure 5.10* as before and then proceed to use the information to decide which of Mr Gibbard's total needs (physiological, security, achievement and self-fulfilment) may be altered for him as an individual at this time. As a guide refer to the sample profiles in Chapter 2, *Figures 2.9, 2.12* and *2.15* and decide how Mr Gibbard is different. Check your ideas with the completed profile, *Figure 5.11*.

**Figure 5.10**   *A patient profile to assist in assessing patients and the development of a problem-solving approach to care*

Name _____ **Mr Gibbard** _____   No. _____

Address _____

Circle any features that are present in your patient in each of the five columns.
Remember that more than one is possible in most of the columns

Section A   1. Starting with the age column, take your selected condition and consider each of the 14 functions requiring assistance and tick in the box(es) those appropriate to your patient's needs, e.g. an elderly patient may require assistance with 2, 3 and 5

Section B   2. Repeat the same procedure with subsequent columns

**(A)  Conditions always present that affect basic needs**

**Physiological disturbances**

| *Age* | *Temperament* | *Social/Cultural* | *Physical/Intellectual Capacity* | Physiological disturbances |
|---|---|---|---|---|
| Newborn | Emotional state or passing mode: | Member of a family unit with friends and status | Normal weight | 1. Fluid and electrolyte imbalance |
| Child | (a) normal | A person relatively alone | Over-weight | 2. Oxygen want |
| Adolescent | (b) euphoric, hyperactive | Maladjusted | Under-weight | 3. Shock |
| Adult | (c) anxious, fearful, agitated, hysterical | Destitute | Normal mentality | 4. Consciousness |
| Middle aged | (d) depressed/ hypoactive | Smoker | Gifted mentality | 5. Local injury/ disease |
| Elderly | | Drinker | Normal sense of: hearing sight equilibrium touch | 6. Metabolism |
| Aged | | | Loss of sense of: hearing sight equilibrium touch | 7. Seeing, hearing, smell and touch |
| | | | Normal motor power | 8. Communicable conditions |
| | | | Loss of motor power | 9. Immobilisation: disease/treatment |

**(B)**

| Functions requiring assistance | Age | Temperament | Social/Cultural | Physical/Intellectual Capacity | Physiological Disturbance |
|---|---|---|---|---|---|
| 1. Breathing | | | | | |
| 2. Eating or drinking | | | | | |
| 3. Elimination | | | | | |
| 4. Sleep or rest | | | | | |
| 5. Movement | | | | | |
| 6. Maintenance of body temperature | | | | | |
| 7. Keeping body clean | | | | | |
| 8. Dressing suitably | | | | | |
| 9. Avoiding dangers and injury | | | | | |
| 10. Communication | | | | | |
| 11. Worship | | | | | |
| 12. Work | | | | | |
| 13. Participation in recreation | | | | | |
| 14. Learning to satisfy curiosity | | | | | |

**Figure 5.11** *Profile for Mr Gibbard*

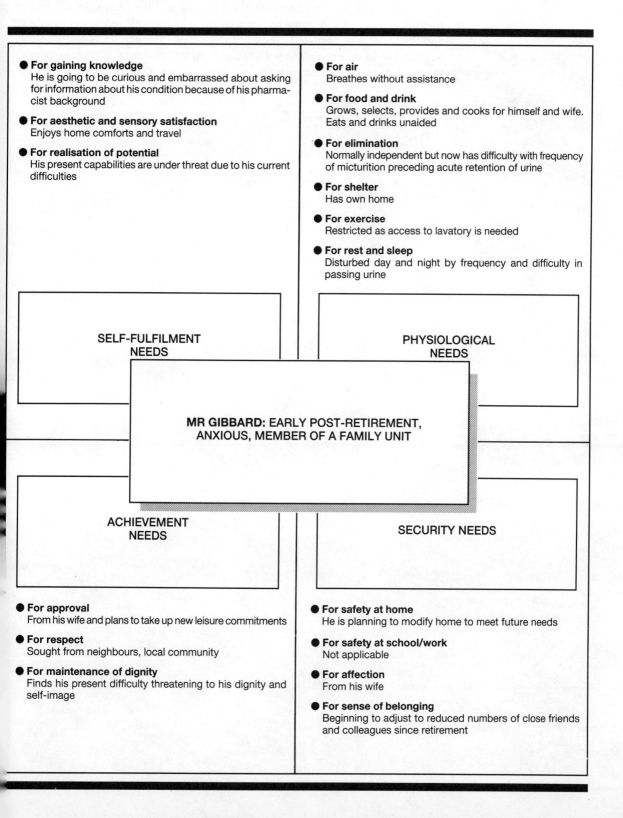

**SELF-FULFILMENT NEEDS**

- **For gaining knowledge**
  He is going to be curious and embarrassed about asking for information about his condition because of his pharmacist background
- **For aesthetic and sensory satisfaction**
  Enjoys home comforts and travel
- **For realisation of potential**
  His present capabilities are under threat due to his current difficulties

**PHYSIOLOGICAL NEEDS**

- **For air**
  Breathes without assistance
- **For food and drink**
  Grows, selects, provides and cooks for himself and wife. Eats and drinks unaided
- **For elimination**
  Normally independent but now has difficulty with frequency of micturition preceding acute retention of urine
- **For shelter**
  Has own home
- **For exercise**
  Restricted as access to lavatory is needed
- **For rest and sleep**
  Disturbed day and night by frequency and difficulty in passing urine

**MR GIBBARD:** EARLY POST-RETIREMENT, ANXIOUS, MEMBER OF A FAMILY UNIT

**ACHIEVEMENT NEEDS**

- **For approval**
  From his wife and plans to take up new leisure commitments
- **For respect**
  Sought from neighbours, local community
- **For maintenance of dignity**
  Finds his present difficulty threatening to his dignity and self-image

**SECURITY NEEDS**

- **For safety at home**
  He is planning to modify home to meet future needs
- **For safety at school/work**
  Not applicable
- **For affection**
  From his wife
- **For sense of belonging**
  Beginning to adjust to reduced numbers of close friends and colleagues since retirement

You are now in a position to complete the lower section of the Assessment Sheet (*Figure 5.10*). Starting with the age column take your selected feature previously circled and consider each of the 14 functions requiring assistance and tick in the box(es) those appropriate to Mr Gibbard's needs. Repeat the same procedure with the subsequent columns. Check your completed Assessment Form with the one that follows, *Figure 5.12*.

**Figure 5.12** *A patient profile to assist in assessing patients and the development of a problem-solving approach to care*

Name __ Mr Gibbard __ No. ____

Address _____

_____

Circle any features that are present in your patient in each of the five columns. Remember that more than one is possible in most of the columns

Section A 1. Starting with the age column, take your selected condition and consider each of the 14 functions requiring assistance and tick in the box(es) those appropriate to your patient's needs, e.g. an elderly patient may require assistance with 2, 3 and 5

Section B 2. Repeat the same procedure with subsequent columns

**(A) Conditions always present that affect basic needs**

**Physiological disturbances**

| Age | Temperament | Social/Cultural | Physical/Intellectual Capacity | Physiological disturbances |
|---|---|---|---|---|
| Newborn | Emotional state | Member of a family | Capacity | 1. Fluid and electrolyte imbalance |
| Child | or passing mode: | unit with friends | Normal weight | 2. Oxygen want |
| Adolescent | (a) normal | and status | Over-weight | 3. Shock |
| Adult | (b) euphoric, | A person relatively | Under-weight | 4. Consciousness |
| Middle aged | hyperactive | alone | Normal mentality | 5. Local injury/disease |
| Elderly | (c) anxious, fearful, | Maladjusted | Gifted mentality | 6. Metabolism |
| Aged | agitated, | Destitute | Normal sense of: | 7. Seeing, hearing, smell and touch |
| | hysterical | Smoker | hearing | 8. Communicable conditions |
| | (d) depressed/ | Drinker | sight | 9. Immobilisation: disease/treatment |
| | hypoactive | | equilibrium | |
| | | | touch | |
| | | | Loss of sense of: | |
| | | | hearing | |
| | | | sight | |
| | | | equilibrium | |
| | | | touch | |
| | | | Normal motor power | |
| | | | Loss of motor power | |

**(B)**

| Functions requiring assistance | Age | Temperament | Social/Cultural | Physical/Intellectual Capacity | Physiological Disturbance |
|---|---|---|---|---|---|
| 1. Breathing | | | | | |
| 2. Eating or drinking | | | | | |
| 3. Elimination | ✓ | | | | ✓ |
| 4. Sleep or rest | ✓ | | | | ✓ |
| 5. Movement | | | | | ✓ |
| 6. Maintenance of body temperature | | | | | |
| 7. Keeping body clean | | | | | |
| 8. Dressing suitably | | | | | ✓ |
| 9. Avoiding dangers and injury | | | | | |
| 10. Communication | ✓ | | | | ✓ |
| 11. Worship | | | | | ✓ |
| 12. Work | | | | | not applicable |
| 13. Participation in recreation | | | | | ✓ |
| 14. Learning to satisfy curiosity | ✓ | | | | ✓ |

You now know that Mr Gibbard's temperament and disease process has a particular effect on his ability to meet his physiological, security, achievement and self-fulfilment needs.

## SELECTING NURSING ACTIONS TO ASSIST A PATIENT WITH DIFFICULTY IN ELIMINATING

The main problem being discussed in this chapter is *difficulty in eliminating* and in this part a patient with difficulty in *micturition*. We would now like you to choose from the list of nursing actions those appropriate for Mr Gibbard by putting a tick in the appropriate column.

Whatever your decision give an explanation for each of your choices and when you have completed this compare your decision and explanations with ours.

Table 5.6    *Nursing action to assist a patient with difficulty in eliminating*

| Nursing actions | Yes | No | Maybe | Reason for choice |
|---|---|---|---|---|
| **Part 1   Breathing** | | | | |
| 1. Provide extra pillows at night | | | | |
| **Part 2   Eating and Drinking** | | | | |
| 1. Offer a normal diet | | | | |
| 2. Offer a high fibre diet | | | | |
| 3. Offer a low residue diet | | | | |
| 4. Offer a fluid diet | | | | |
| 5. Offer a high protein diet | | | | |
| 6. Encourage patient to drink hourly | | | | |
| 7. Advise patient to restrict amount of fluid drunk | | | | |
| 8. Discover likes and dislikes | | | | |
| 9. Assist in completing menu requests | | | | |
| **Part 3   Eliminating** | | | | |
| 1. Give suppositories | | | | |
| 2. Give an enema | | | | |
| 3. Give an aperient | | | | |
| 4. Allow patient to go to toilet as required using a bedpan or urinal | | | | |
| 5. Offer bedpan as required | | | | |

*Table 5.6    Continued*

| Nursing actions | Yes | No | Maybe | Reason for choice |
|---|---|---|---|---|
| **Part 3 Eliminating (continued)** | | | | |
| 6. Offer commode day or night | | | | |
| 7. Perform manual evacuation | | | | |
| 8. Give rectal/colon washouts | | | | |
| 9. Prepare patient for sigmoidoscopy biopsy and/ or barium enema | | | | |
| 10. Check function by urinary drainage apparatus | | | | |
| 11. Check catheter entry site for sepsis | | | | |
| **Part 4    Sleeping and Resting** | | | | |
| 1. Offer warm drink at night | | | | |
| 2. Ensure adequate ventilation in the ward | | | | |
| 3. Position patient's bed near to the toilet | | | | |
| 4. Position patient's bed at top end of ward away from toilets | | | | |
| 5. Offer night sedation | | | | |
| **Part 5    Moving** | | | | |
| 1. Keep patient at complete rest | | | | |
| 2. Encourage exercise | | | | |
| 3. Sit in easy chair | | | | |
| 4. Assist in repositioning in bed | | | | |
| 5. Provide a sheepskin | | | | |
| 6. Provide a ripple bed | | | | |
| 7. Provide a hoist | | | | |
| **Part 6    Maintaining Body Temperature** | | | | |
| 1. Provide plenty of blankets | | | | |
| 2. Provide light bed clothes | | | | |
| **Part 7    Keeping Body Clean** | | | | |
| 1. Give daily bedbath | | | | |
| 2. Assist patient washing in bed | | | | |

*Table 5.6    Continued*

| Nursing actions | Yes | No | Maybe | Reason for choice |
|---|---|---|---|---|
| **Part 7 Keeping Body Clean (continued)** | | | | |
| 3. Assist patient washing in bathroom | | | | |
| 4. Encourage patient to bath | | | | |
| 5. Assist patient to shave and brush hair | | | | |
| 6. Provide opportunity to wash after eliminating | | | | |
| 7. Offer antiseptic mouthwashes | | | | |
| 8. Give oral toilet | | | | |
| **Part 8   Dressing Suitably** | | | | |
| 1. Provide hospital pyjamas | | | | |
| 2. Provide hospital dressing gown and slippers | | | | |
| 3. Encourage use of own pyjamas | | | | |
| 4. Encourage to be up and dressed during the day | | | | |
| 5. Provide aids to prevent soiling of clothing | | | | |
| **Part 9   Avoiding Dangers and Injury** | | | | |
| 1. Provide facilities for adequate hand washing after eliminating | | | | |
| **Part 10   Communicating** | | | | |
| 1. Allocate a nurse to the patient | | | | |
| 2. Assist in contact with relatives | | | | |
| 3. Give an opportunity for exchange of information with patient, relatives and staff | | | | |
| 4. Encourage him to participate in conversation with staff | | | | |
| 5. Position patient's bed in the middle of the ward to promote social interaction | | | | |
| 6. Position patient's bed in a side ward to provide privacy | | | | |
| 7. Make an appointment for stoma therapist to visit | | | | |
| **Part 11   Worshipping** | | | | |
| 1. Inform hospital chaplain | | | | |

*Table 5.6    Continued*

| Nursing actions | Yes | No | Maybe | Reason for choice |
|---|---|---|---|---|
| **Part 11 Worshipping (continued)** | | | | |
| 2. Inform patient's own chaplain of patient's admission | | | | |
| 3. Ignore spiritual needs until patient is feeling better | | | | |
| **Part 12    Working** | | | | |
| Not appropriate as patient is retired and not in permanent employment | | | | |
| **Part 13    Participating in Recreation** | | | | |
| 1. Provide formal occupational therapy | | | | |
| 2. Assist patient in using the television room | | | | |
| **Part 14    Learning to Satisfy Curiosity** | | | | |
| 1. Keep patient fully informed of condition and progress | | | | |
| 2. Avoid discussing problems in eliminating | | | | |

## EXPLANATION FOR CHOICE OF NURSING ACTIONS

### Part 1    Breathing

You should have ticked the Maybe column. Mr Gibbard may find it more comfortable to breathe sitting up if bladder is distended.

### Part 2    Eating and Drinking

You should have ticked in the Yes column numbers 1, 6 and 8. We would expect Mr Gibbard to enjoy a normal diet taking account of his likes and dislikes. He will need encouragement to drink as he knows he has difficulty in passing urine and may be reluctant to drink.

You should have ticked numbers 2 and 9 in the Maybe column; a high fibre diet helps to stimulate the bowel and produce regular bowel actions without straining the rectum, and the pelvic cavity is kept relatively empty of faeces and defaecation can stimulate micturition. Help may be offered to select high fibre foods. You should have ticked numbers 3, 4 and 5 in the No column. None of these are appropriate for the reasons given above.

### Part 3    Eliminating

You should have ticked in the Yes column numbers 4, 10 and 11: number 4 to enable him to maintain normal bowel activity and numbers 10 and 11 for maintaining his urinary output in the present state. You could have ticked the Maybe column for numbers 1, 3, 5 and 6. Suppositories and aperient may be necessary to assist him in emptying the lower bowel. Numbers 5 and 6 are dependent on his capabilities and degree of difficulty with micturition. The No column should have been used for numbers 2, 7, 8 and 9. None of these are appropriate for this patient.

### Part 4   Sleeping and Resting

Numbers 1, 2 and 3 should be in the Yes column. Numbers 1 and 2 can assist in settling and provide comfort to the patient. Number 3 should be ticked in the Yes column as the patient should be able to reach the toilet without having to go far and to disturb other patients. Number 4 should be in the No column for the opposite reason to number 3. Number 5, night sedation, could be helpful in assisting Mr Gibbard to get adequate sleep and rest.

### Part 5   Moving

We hope you have ticked numbers 2 and 3 in the Yes column as we would wish to maintain his present mobility and independence. If he is weak, then you should have ticked the Maybe column for numbers 4, 5 and 7 by helping him to reposition himself in bed and with the use of a sheepskin and hoist you would assist in preventing the risks of bedrest. The No column should be ticked for numbers 1 and 6 as neither are appropriate for Mr Gibbard at this time. Care of bladder drainage when moving is necessary to prevent kinking or traction on the tubing. The apparatus should be discreetly carried when walking to avoid embarrassment and loss of dignity.

### Part 6   Maintaining Body Temperature

You should have ticked the Maybe column for both the actions which are dependent on personal preference and environmental temperature.

### Part 7   Keeping Body Clean

We hope you have ticked the Yes column for numbers 4, 5 and 6. Encouraging the patient to bath himself, shave and brush his hair maintains some independence, and provision of washing facilities following elimination assists in prevention of cross-infection. You should have ticked numbers 2 and 3 in the Maybe column as assistance may be required at the bedside or in the bathroom. You should have considered using the No column for numbers 1, 7 and 8. These are not appropriate for Mr Gibbard at this time.

### Part 8   Dressing Suitably

You should have ticked the Yes column for numbers 3 and 5. Mr Gibbard may need aids to prevent soiling due to leakage from drainage tube. You could have ticked the Maybe column for numbers 1, 2 and 4 although these will depend on Mr Gibbard's preferences and degree of difficulty.

### Part 9   Avoiding Dangers and Injury

You should have ticked the Yes column here because of the risk of cross infection to other patients and staff.

### Part 10 Communicating

We hope you have ticked the Yes column for numbers 1, 2, 3 and 4 to assist in developing communication links between patient, staff and relatives. Numbers 5 and 6 should be ticked in the Maybe column as this would be dependent on his wishes and the facilities available. Number 7 is not applicable to Mr Gibbard.

### Part 11 Worshipping

Items 1 and 2 could have been ticked in the Maybe column if and whichever the patient wishes. Number 3 should be in the No column; if acknowledged by the patient spiritual needs should be met promptly.

### Part 12 Working

Mr Gibbard is retired therefore this section is not appropriate.

### Part 13 Participating in Recreation

You should have ticked the Maybe column for number 2 as Mr Gibbard may need assistance. Number 1 should be No: formal occupational therapy is not appropriate for Mr Gibbard at this time.

### Part 14 Learning to Satisfy Curiosity

You should have ticked Yes for number 1, as he should be kept informed even though he may not appear to be questioning about his condition. Item 2 should have been ticked in the No column. He has difficulty with elimination and should be encouraged to verbalise his fears and anxieties on what could be a difficult subject.

You can now see that some of these nursing actions are dependent on the individual characteristics of Mr Gibbard and therefore his care plan needs to be sensitive to his individual needs. However, Mr Gibbard's difficulty is with micturition and should therefore have similar priorities in nursing actions as for Mr Lewis who had difficulty with defaecation. Both are problems associated with eliminating.

Return to *Table 5.4* and read again to see whether you agree with the priorities. If you wish to remind yourself about planning and providing nursing care, refer again to *Table 3.4*.

### IDENTIFICATION OF CRITERIA FOR PROGRESS

You should now read carefully the plan shown in *Table 5.7* for identifying criteria for progress.

Table 5.7   *Plan of care for progress*

| Nursing actions to assist a patient with difficulty in micturition | Yes | Maybe | Priority Choice | Measurements | Short-term goals | Review period | Evaluation Criteria Have short-term goals been met? |
|---|---|---|---|---|---|---|---|
| **Part 3   Eliminating** | | | | Record: Urinary drainage via supra-pubic catheter | Ensure patency of urinary drainage | On-going | Continues |
| 1. Give suppositories | | ✔ | | | | | |
| 3. Give an aperient | | ✔ | | Check: functioning of the urinary drainage system | Output of 2–2½ litres of clear sterile urine | 8-hourly | Since initial emptying of bladder, has drained 1000 ml only |
| 4. Allow patient to go to toilet as required using a bedpan or urinal | ✔ | | | Note: (a) Presence of blood in the urine | | | (a) No blood in urine |
| 5. Offer bedpan as required | | ✔ | FIRST | (b) Abdominal pain or pain around catheter entry site | Pain free and wound clean | On-going | (b)One episode of abdominal pain when tube became blocked due to kinking |
| 6. Offer commode day or night | | ✔ | | (c) Anxiety or agitation | Relaxed, not agitated | On-going | (c)Naturally became anxious when blockage and pain occurred |
| 10. Check functions of urinary drainage apparatus | ✔ | | | Obtain: (a) Sample of urine for culture and sensitivity, cytology | (a) For medical assessment and decision regarding cystoscopy and further treatment | (a) When results available | (a) Awaiting results |
| 11. Check catheter entry site for sepsis | ✔ | | | (b) Assist with obtaining blood samples for urea, electrolytes, haemoglobin and full blood count | | | (b) Blood test results within normal limits |
| | | | | Record: Frequency and nature of bowel actions | Normal evacuation | 24-hourly | Suppositories necessary, then bowel action normal |

*Table 5.7 Continued*

| Nursing actions to assist a patient with difficulty in micturition | Yes | Maybe | Priority Choice | Measurements | Short-term goals | Review period | Evaluation Criteria Have short-term goals been met? |
|---|---|---|---|---|---|---|---|
| **Part 2 Eating and Drinking**<br><br>1. Offer a normal diet<br><br>2. Offer a high fibre diet<br><br>6. Encourage patient to drink hourly<br><br>8. Discover likes and dislikes<br><br>9. Assist in completing menu requests | ✓<br><br><br>✓<br>✓ | <br><br>✓<br><br><br><br><br><br>✓ | SECOND | Record:<br>(a) The amount of food eaten and fluid drunk<br><br>(b) Frequency of taking food and drink<br><br>(c) When he feels hungry<br><br>(d) Type of intake, likes and dislikes<br><br>(e) Weight | (a), (b), (c), (d) Intake of 3 litres of fluid and 2000 calories in 24 hours<br><br><br><br><br>(e) Provide a baseline for surgery | (a) (b) (d) 8-hourly<br><br><br><br>(c) 24-hourly<br><br>Prior to discharge | During 1st 24 hours drunk 1500 ml only<br><br>Consumed 1500 calories<br><br><br><br>Weight: 70 kg |
| **Part 4 Sleeping and Resting**<br><br>1. Offer warm drink at night<br><br>2. Ensure adequate ventilation in the ward<br><br>3. Position patient's bed near the toilet<br><br>5. Offer night sedation<br><br>**Part 1 Breathing**<br><br>1. Provide extra pillows at night | ✓<br><br>✓<br><br>✓ | <br><br><br><br><br><br>✓<br><br><br><br>✓ | THIRD | Record:<br>(a) Length of sleep<br><br>(b) Number of times disturbed during the night and why<br><br>(c) Whether night sedation is required | 6–7 hours undisturbed sleep or rest | 24 hourly (am) | Disturbed once during the night due to abdominal pain from blocked drainage tube. Night sedation not required |
| **Part 10 Communicating**<br><br>1. Allocate a nurse to the patient<br><br>2. Assist in contact with relatives<br><br>3. Give an opportunity for exchange of information with patient, relatives and staff<br><br>4. Encourage him to participate in conversation with staff | ✓<br><br>✓<br><br><br>✓<br><br><br><br>✓ | | FOURTH | Note levels of anxiety and frustration from patient and relatives | Mr Gibbard is content with care being given and feels able to relate to staff | On-going | Mr Gibbard's wife is visiting daily<br><br>Medical staff have discussed progress and plan of treatment with both Mr and Mrs Gibbard. Advised to consider delaying his departure for the USA |

*Table 5.7   Continued*

| Nursing actions to assist a patient with difficulty in micturition. | Yes | Maybe | Priority Choice | Measurements | Short-term goals | Review period | Evaluation Criteria Have short-term goals been met? |
|---|---|---|---|---|---|---|---|
| **Part 10 Communicating (continued)** | | | | | | | Wife in contact with local church |
| 5. Position patient's bed in the middle of the ward to promote social interaction | | ✓ | | | | | |
| 6. Position patient's bed in a side ward to provide privacy | | ✓ | FOURTH | | | | |
| **Part 11   Worshipping** | | | | | | | |
| 1. Inform hospital chaplain | | ✓ | | | | | |
| 2. Inform patient's own chaplain of his admission | | ✓ | | | | | |
| **Part 14   Learning to Satisfy Curiosity** | | | | | | | |
| 1. Keep patient fully informed of condition and progress | ✓ | | | | | | |
| **Part 9   Avoiding Dangers and Injury** | | | FIFTH | Note whether Mr Gibbard is attentive to personal hygiene | Minimise risk of cross-infection | On-going | Mr Gibbard is fastidious about personal hygiene |
| 1. Provide facilities for adequate hand washing after eliminating | ✓ | | | | | | |
| **Part 5   Moving** | | | SIXTH | Note level of activity. Check that tubing is not kinked or pulled and is discreetly carried | Adequate rest to compensate for disturbances. Is not embarrassed by apparatus | 24-hourly | Up for most of the afternoon after resting in the morning |
| 2. Encourage exercise | ✓ | | | | | | |
| 3. Sit in easy chair | ✓ | | | | | | |
| 4. Assist in repositioning in bed | | ✓ | | | | | |
| 5. Provide a sheepskin | | ✓ | | | | | |
| 7. Provide a hoist | | ✓ | | | | | |
| **Part 6   Maintaining Body Temperature** | | | | Record body temperature twice a day | Body temperature to remain within normal limits | 12-hourly | No rise in temperature |
| 1. Provide plenty of blankets | | ✓ | | | | | |
| 2. Provide light bed clothes | | ✓ | | | | | |

*Table 5.7    Continued*

| Nursing actions to assist a patient with difficulty in micturition. | Yes | Maybe | Priority Choice | Measurements | Short-term goals | Review period | Evaluation Criteria Have short-term goals been met? |
|---|---|---|---|---|---|---|---|
| **Part 8    Dressing Suitably** | | | SIXTH | Check discreetly for soiling | Minimise any loss of dignity and independence | 8-hourly | No leakage, managing to cope with drainage apparatus |
| 1. Provide hospital pyjamas | | ✓ | | | | | |
| 2. Provide hospital dressing gown | | ✓ | | | | | |
| 3. Encourage use of own pyjamas | ✓ | | | | | | |
| 4. Encourage to be up and dressed during the day | | ✓ | | | | | |
| 5. Provide aids to prevent soiling of clothes | ✓ | | | | | | |
| **Part 13    Participating in Recreation** | | | SEVENTH | Note Mr Gibbard's interest in outside affairs | Prevent boredom and brooding about present condition | On-going | Watches the news on television. Attention span short |
| 2. Assist patient in using the television room | | ✓ | | | | | |

### Using Evaluation Criteria for Resetting Short-term Goals

We would like to suggest that you reconsider Mr Gibbard's evaluation criteria at the end of his first 24 hours in hospital and decide on new priorities for nursing actions, revised measurements and setting new short-term goals for preparing him for cytoscopy and surgical intervention (prostatectomy).

### IDENTIFICATION OF LONG-TERM GOALS

We would expect that after surgery Mr Gibbard would be able to return home and maintain his health, and be confident that he can obtain guidance from his GP as required. If you look at the individual profile prepared for Mr Gibbard on admission to hospital in this chapter and the individual profiles numbers 9 and 15 in Chapter 2, Section 1, you can complete a long-term goal profile which will indicate his expected level of independence for his age and social setting.

## REFERENCES, FURTHER READING AND TECHNIQUES

### References

Boore, J. (1980). Normal and abnormal micturition, *Nursing (Oxford)*, **18**, pages 763–765.

Green, J. H. *Basic Clinical Physiology*, 3rd edition. OUP, Oxford.

Hunt, P and Sendell, B. (1987). *Nursing the Adult with a Specific Physiological Disturbance*, 2nd edition. Macmillan Education, London.

Tierney, A. (1980). Toilet training the mentally handicapped, *Nursing (Oxford)*, pages 795–797.

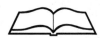

### *Suggested Further Reading*

*Related to Medical Conditions Affecting Eliminating*

Macleod, J. (Ed.) *Davidson's Principles and Practice of Medicine*, 13th edition. Churchill Livingstone, Edinburgh, 1983: Chapter 5 pp. 127–144; Chapter 8 pp. 359–375; Chapter 10 pp. 421–457; Chapter 17 pp. 792–895.

Read, A. E., Barritt, D. W. and Hewer, R. *Modern Medicine*, 3rd edition. Pitman Medical, London, 1984: Chapter 5 pp. 82–109; Chapter 16 pp. 261–297; Chapter 17 pp. 298–308; Chapter 24 pp. 638–660.

These references include:
- Conditions of the lower bowel
- Conditions of the urinary system
- Disorders of water and electrolytes
- Conditions found in tropical countries

*Related to Surgical Conditions Affecting Eliminating*

Ellis, H. and Wastell, C. *Surgery for Nurses*. Blackwell Scientific, Oxford, 1980: Chapters 12–15 pp. 198–368.

Henderson, M. A. *Essential Surgery for Nurses*. Churchill Livingstone, Edinburgh, 1980: Chapters 23–27 pp. 111–141; Chapters 35–37 pp. 181–208.

Horton, R. *General Surgery and the Nurse*. Hodder and Stoughton, London, 1983: Chapters 16–20 pp. 139–197; Chapters 24–26 pp. 235–262.

These references include:

*Defaecation*
The small intestine:
- Meckel's diverticulum
- Crohn's disease
- Tumours
- Obstruction
- Strangulated hernia

The appendix
Peritonitis
The large colon
- Diverticulitis
- Tumours
- Colostomy

The rectum and anal area
- Ano-rectal atresia
- Hirschsprung's disease
- Haemorrhoids
- Fistula-in-ano
- Carcinoma of rectum
Herniae

*Micturition*
Trauma affecting the urinary tract
Calculi
Tumours of the kidney and bladder
Ruptured urethra
Stricture of the urethra
Prostatic enlargement
Carcinoma of the prostate gland
Urinary retention
Phimosis

### Pharmacology Related to Care of Patients with Difficulty in Micturition

You may wish to familiarise yourself with the medicines commonly used for patients with difficulty in *micturition*.

Muscle relaxants
Urinary antibiotics

### Suggested Nursing Procedures / Guidelines for Nursing Practice

You may wish to familiarise yourself with your local policies and procedures/ guidelines for nursing practice which may be applicable to a patient requiring assistance with difficulty in *micturition*. Here is a suggested list:

- Aseptic technique
- Bladder irrigation
- Catheter:
  emptying urinary bag
  urethral insertion
  urine specimen collection
  indwelling, care of and removal
  suprapubic, insertion and removal

# Chapter 6
# Sleeping and Resting

## NORMAL PHYSIOLOGY

Before proceeding we suggest you revise your knowledge of the central nervous system by using the following references and text.

- Hunt and Sendell (1987). *Nursing the Adult with a Specific Physiological Disturbance*, 2nd edn.
- Green (1978). *Basic Clinical Physiology*, pages 129–152.

## SLEEPING

### The Concept of Sleep

Sleep is a period of loss of consciousness which affects everybody every day but can be distinguished from unconsciousness as it is possible to be roused by shouts of 'Fire', and by telephone and alarms ringing. This demonstrates that some kind of 'watching guard' is maintained by the higher cortex of the brain while we go 'off duty'.

### Length of Sleep

Age affects the amount of sleep a person needs. For babies it can be as long as 16 hours with 6–8 periods of sleep throughout the 24 hours. This gradually consolidates into longer periods of sleep and wakefulness and begins to occupy the night hours rather than the day. By the age of 4 years children can sleep about 11 hours per night with a short daytime nap, but by 5 years this is no required. By the age of 15 years, 7 to 8 hours of sleep is being taken and this continues to the age of about 60 years.

From the age of 40 years until retirement sleep tends to become slightly longer and more broken. During old age the sleep pattern can return to rapid alternation between sleep and wakefulness, rather like children under one year of age.

### Long and Short Sleepers

People vary in the length of sleep they require and there is little to prove whether long or short sleepers are psychologically healthier. If we want to sleep longer we usually have to go to bed earlier because the pressures of everyday life keep us keyed to a 24-hour day rather than wanting to go to bed when we require sleep.

### Sleep Deprivation

There appears to be a need for sleep and if kept awake people can suffer from lack of concentration and a prolonged response to stimulus. In extreme sleep deprivation bizarre hallucinations can be experienced.

### Normal Sleep

When we prepare for sleep we turn off the light and adopt a favourite sleeping position, for example, curled up, flat on back or lying on one side. We close our eyes and within a few minutes start to doze. During this time our mind wanders and we drift in and out of sleep without realising it. We can easily be disturbed by the slightest touch, draught or creak. We can have no memory of this time and can deny that we have slept at all. Within 30 minutes we enter sleep proper, the body relaxes, the heart beats slow and body position changes are slow. We are unaware of things around us but can be awakened by a *new* sound.

The deepest stage of sleep is reached after one hour when heartbeat and breathing are slow and we appear 'dead to the world'. During this time we can ignore all outside stimulation and can be extremely difficult to wake. If we are disturbed, it can take time to wake up completely and we are often irrational in our responses. Brain waves are measurements of the electrical activity of the brain cells and are normally fast, small in amplitude and desynchronised during wakefulness. They become slow and synchronised during sleep. They are at their slowest during deep sleep and continue for about 30 minutes when the deepest stage of sleep has been reached.

After this the waves begin to speed up and sleep becomes lighter. Breathing and heart rate increases and body position is changed more frequently. During this phase we will probably open our eyes and look from side to side as if seeing something. This is commonly called REM (rapid eye movement) sleep. We can become sexually roused, dream, experience a nightmare and be difficult to rouse. This period lasts for about 15 minutes.

This cycle of deep sleep, light sleep and REM sleep repeats itself about four times in an eight-hour sleep period.

## RESTING

Resting is a period of cessation of activity, a letting go of body and mind. The body is relaxed, the heart rate and breathing are slowed, a comfortable position is adopted but unlike sleep, consciousness is not lost. During the course of the day and during waking periods at night the body can be rested, allowing recharging of energy and refreshment.

### Relaxation Aids

Some aids to relaxation are outlined in *Figure 6.1*.

**Figure 6.1**    *Resting*

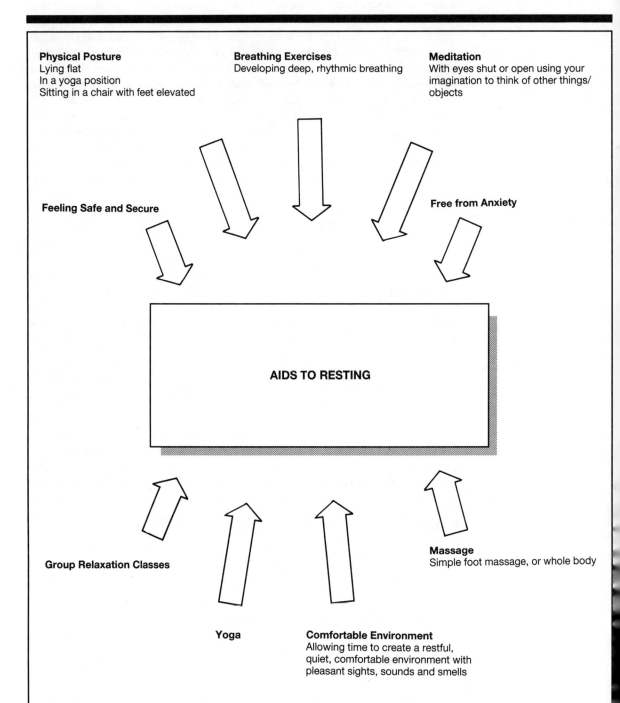

**Physical Posture**
Lying flat
In a yoga position
Sitting in a chair with feet elevated

**Breathing Exercises**
Developing deep, rhythmic breathing

**Meditation**
With eyes shut or open using your imagination to think of other things/objects

**Feeling Safe and Secure**

**Free from Anxiety**

**AIDS TO RESTING**

**Group Relaxation Classes**

**Massage**
Simple foot massage, or whole body

**Yoga**

**Comfortable Environment**
Allowing time to create a restful, quiet, comfortable environment with pleasant sights, sounds and smells

## SOCIOLOGICAL FACTORS AFFECTING SLEEPING AND RESTING

Sleeping and resting is affected by the environment we live in and the health and age of the individuals in society. Sleeping and resting appears to occur more easily if free from excessive and sudden noises, such as heavy traffic noise, thunder, doors banging or sirens sounding. Sleep can be disturbed by bright, flashing lights such as traffic lights, neon signs or flashes of lightning. Bright sunlight can disturb night workers who are trying to sleep during the day. Smells can also disturb sleep and rest and common causes can be smoke, refuse, industrial complexes, farmyards or sewage farms. Crowded and/or public sleeping areas can inhibit sleep such as in hostels, hospital wards, campsites, overcrowded housing and shared beds in large families. Some individuals may be more susceptible to sleeping difficulties because of their age (e.g. the young adult and the elderly sleep less) and their general state of health. Some medical conditions may directly affect sleeping such as thyrotoxicosis, acute anxiety states. The susceptibility of the individual and the environmental factors affecting sleeping and resting can be considered as before on a 10 point scale.

### Interrelationship of Environmental Factors and the Vulnerability of the Individual

On the following chart (*Figure 6.2*) we would like you to insert an X using the two scales from the following examples.

*Mr Davidson* is a fit 35-year-old and is married with no children. He lives with his wife in a small semi-detached house in a quiet cul-de-sac in a city suburb. He works a five-day week in a local bank and belongs to the nearby social and sports club. He relaxes by watching television and reading.

Scale 2   Vulnerability
Scale 1   Environment

*Miss Susan Cotton*, aged 25 years, lives in the top flat in a multi-occupied old Victorian house in a city and her bedroom window is in close proximity to a newly built motorway flyover. She is disturbed by the noise of the traffic and the smell of exhaust fumes. Despite having heavy curtains she finds the irregular movement of car headlights a hindrance to her sleep.

Scale 2   Vulnerability
Scale 9   Environment

*Mr Joseph* lives in a secluded country cottage by a stream. He is active in countryside pursuits which he uses for relaxation, and particularly enjoys fishing. Despite these pleasant surroundings Mr Joseph has found that since retiring from his job as a farmworker he seems to sleep only intermittently and for less length of time at night, and requires a rest period after lunch.

Scale 8   Vulnerability
Scale 2   Environment

*Mrs Wootten*, aged 80 years, is in hospital recovering from pneumonia and hopes to be discharged in a few days time to her Warden controlled flat. The ward admits 4 to 6 acutely ill patients every 24 hours. Mrs Wootten's bed is near the nurses' station and utility rooms.

Scale 9   Vulnerability
Scale 10  Environment

**Figure 6.2**   *Chart to illustrate the interrelationships of environment and the vulnerability of the individual.*

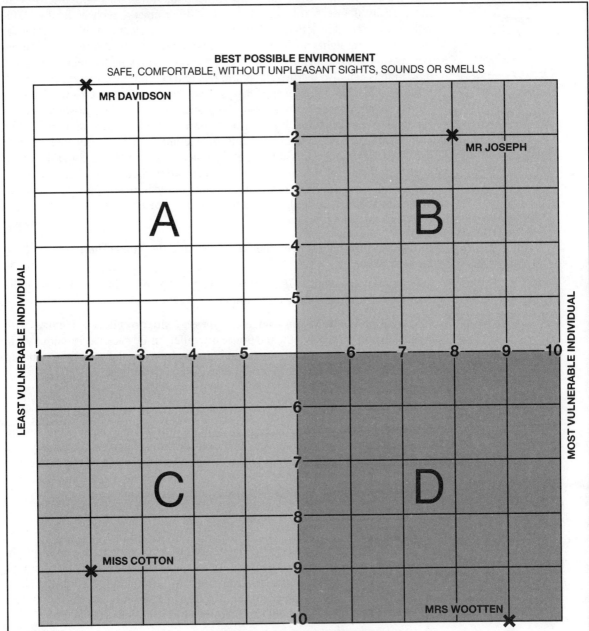

You can now see into which sections the different individuals fit. Mr Davidson is in Section A: as a fit adult in a suitable environment, he is at little risk of having sleeping and resting difficulties. Mr Joseph and Miss Cotton are in Sections B and C, respectively. Mr Joseph is most at risk because his age makes him vulnerable, while Miss Cotton is at most risk due to her environment.

Miss Wootten is at high risk: she is the most vulnerable because of her age and ill health and also because of being in the worst environment for sleeping and resting. She is disturbed by being in a public place, by the strange, irregular noises, unpleasant smells and lights. The constant activity around her bedside is potentially threatening to her sense of security.

The measures outlined in *Figures 6.3* and *6.4* can help to improve the environment for sleeping and resting and reduce the vulnerability of the individual.

**Figure 6.3**   *Factors which help to improve the environment for sleeping and resting*

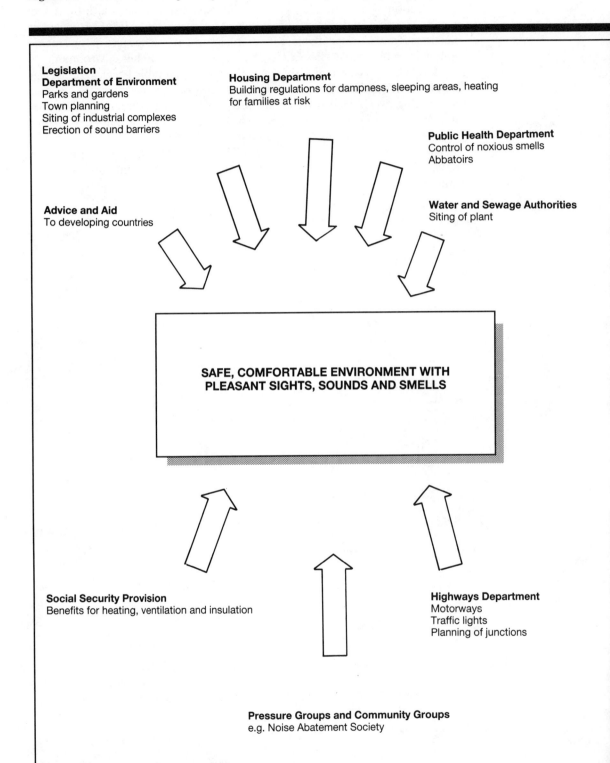

**Figure 6.4** *Factors which help to reduce the vulnerabilty of the individual*

**Health Care provision**
For vulnerable groups
For the sick and unhealthy

**Health Education Council**
Advice to parents on child's sleep
requirements
Preparation for retirement and
changing patterns of sleep
Use and abuse of sedatives and
narcotics
Prevention of unsuitable aids to
relaxation, e.g. cannabis, alcohol

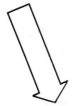
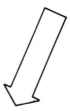

**REDUCE THE VULNERABILITY
OF THE INDIVIDUAL**

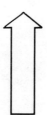

**Aids to sleep and rest**
Meditation
Breathing exercises
Yoga
Group relaxation classes

PSYCHOLOGICAL FACTORS AFFECTING SLEEPING AND RESTING

**Figure 6.5**   *Some psychological factors affecting sleeping and resting*

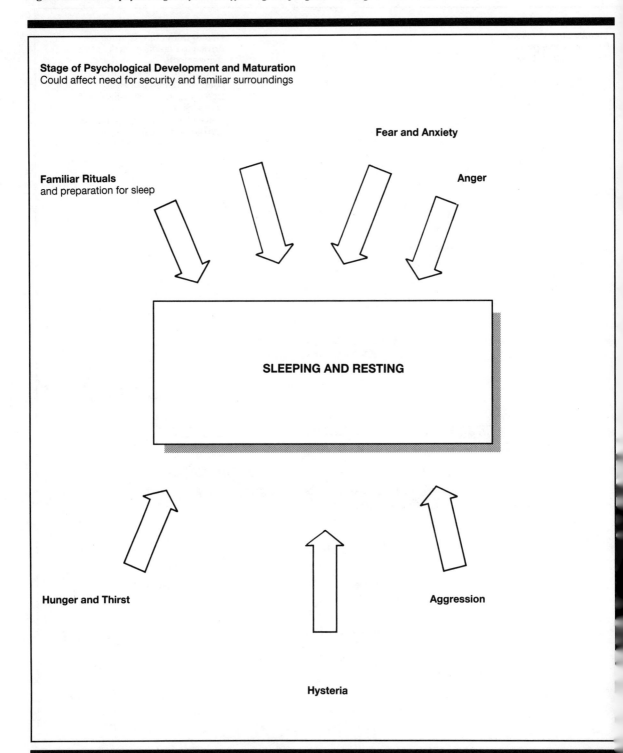

## PATIENT HISTORY

We would now like to consider a patient who has difficulty in sleeping and resting. While you are reading Miss Scott's history it is important to bear in mind the effects of the environment and the vulnerability of Miss Scott. The clinical features of inadequate sleep and rest are explained in *Table 6.1* but you should note that the clinical features of thyrotoxicosis are not discussed here. These can be found in Hunt and Sendell (1983) pages 152 and 170.

Miss Josephine Scott, aged 40 years, is a floor supervisor in a well-known department store. She owns a flat on a small development site and is involved in local community affairs including the local ratepayers association and photographic society. Once a month she visits her parents who live in the next county. About eighteen months ago she visited her GP complaining of:

● Loss of weight despite increased appetite
● Sweating of face and hands
● Intolerance of heat
● Irritability with colleagues at work

Following discussions and examination the doctor found:

● An anxious, talkative, active person
● Skin moist, hair lank and greasy
● Pulse rate rapid
● Temperature and blood pressure normal
● Fine tremor of hands
● Slight exophthalmos
● Slightly enlarged thyroid gland (goitre)

He suspected an over-active thyroid gland and made arrangements for Miss Scott to attend the local medical outpatient's department for further investigations. These included blood tests such as total serum thyroxine, serum thyroid stimulating hormone levels in response to thyroid releasing hormone stimulation; and an electrocardiogram.

The results confirmed a diagnosis of thyrotoxicosis with no evidence of heart involvement and the doctor discussed with her the alternative treatments of antithyroid drug therapy and surgery. He explained that medical treatment, though prolonged, could be entirely successful, but if unsuccessful, surgery could be contemplated later.

He prescribed carbimazole 15 mg three times a day for 4 weeks, and then a reduced maintenance dose giving as little as possible to achieve a euthyroid state. He explained to her that she must report any sore throat or any other infection as it is important to stop this drug immediately and give antibiotics as carbimazole can damage the bone marrow and reduce the normal response to infection. He told her that it would take several weeks for any noticeable effect but she should start to regain weight, her appetite should return to normal and she should begin to feel less irritable and sweaty. Over the next 18 months Miss Scott improved initially but 2 months ago she started to get recurrence of her original symptoms. Her doctor advised that she should be admitted to hospital for partial thyroidectomy. In the interim he increased the dosage of carbimazole and explained that this would be discontinued 10 days prior to operation when she would be given Lugol's iodine three times a day.

## EXPLANATION OF CLINICAL FEATURES

*Table 6.1.  Explanation of difficulties in sleeping and resting*

| Normal physiology | Abnormal physiology | Clinical features |
|---|---|---|
| The production and release of thyroxine from the thyroid gland is dependent on:<br>(a) Intake and absorption of iodine in the diet<br>(b) Thyroid-stimulating hormone from the anterior pituitary gland<br><br>(c) Normal functioning thyroid cells | (a) Intake and absorption of iodine is normal<br>(b) Thyroid-stimulating hormone levels are reduced but LATS (long-acting thyroid stimulators) often present<br>(c) Thyroid cells become over-active and secrete constant high levels of thyroxine | (c) The enlarged gland can cause pressure on the trachea which may only be obvious when sleeping in certain positions. Patient may wake with feeling of distress or suffocation |
| Control of serum levels of thyroxine is by feedback mechanism on the pituitary gland | Feedback mechanism control is lost and gland enlarges | |
| Thyroxine acts in the following ways:<br>(a) It controls the rate of utilisation of oxygen by the tissue cells (metabolic rate)<br><br>(b) It is necessary for normal function of the nervous system<br><br><br><br><br><br><br><br><br><br>(c) It is necessary for healthy skin, hair and mental activity<br>(d) It is necessary for normal red blood cell production | (a) Excessive thyroxine increases rate of oxygen utilisation resulting in increased respirations and pulse rate; loss of weight with increased appetite<br>(b) Excess causes over-excitability and nervousness. Effects on autonomic nervous system cause tachycardia, diarrhoea, palor and sweating. Excessive sympathetic activity can cause the eyeballs to protrude by pulling on the muscles of the upper eyelid exposing more of the eyeball than usual. In some patients exophthalmos may also be due to deposition of excess fat in the orbit behind the eye<br>(c) Excess thyroxine causes greasy skin and hair and irritability<br>(d) Unchanged in thyrotoxicosis | (a) Heart rate and respiration remain elevated at sleep<br><br>(b) Difficult to relax, disturbed excessively by outside stimuli and hunger, sleeps for short periods only. Restless<br><br><br><br><br><br><br><br><br><br>(c) Awakes tired and irritable |

## Special Note

We would like to point out that this chapter gives consideration to the care required for a patient with sleeping and resting difficulties. We look at the ways sleeping and resting difficulties affect living activities, but for clarity, any other problems related to Miss Scott and her illness will not be considered when we come to the selection of Nursing Actions. You must, therefore, bear in mind that this is an incomplete plan of care devised to emphasise the *subject of this chapter only*.

## EFFECTS OF DIFFICULTY OF SLEEPING AND RESTING ON OTHER LIVING ACTIVITIES

Most people seem to benefit physically and mentally from sleep and rest. It can assist the individual to meet physiological, safety, achievement and self-fulfilment needs. If a person has difficulty in sleeping and resting most of the living activities can be affected.

### Difficulty in Sleeping and Resting

1. *Breathing*
   Not affected.

2. *Eating and Drinking*
   With general tiredness may lack energy to select, provide, cook and eat and drink food and fluids.

3. *Eliminating*
   Upsets normal routine and habits.

4. *Sleeping and Resting*
   Difficulty in settling, altered length and depth of sleep. Exhausted on waking.

5. *Moving*
   Reduced due to lack of energy.

6. *Maintaining Body Temperature*
   Temperature may alter due to excessive restlessness.

7. *Keeping Body Clean*
   Reduced attention to detail as too weary.

8. *Dressing Suitably*
   Reduced attention to detail as too weary.

9. *Avoiding Danger and Injury*
   Less attentive to hazards as too weary.

10. *Communicating*
    Can become irritable and/or withdrawn as a result of lack of sleep and want to talk about little else.

11. *Worshipping*
    Could be too tired to make the effort to attend public worship.

12. *Working*
    Could fail to arrive for work on time. Inattentive to detail at work.

13. *Participating in Recreation*
    May choose inappropriate recreation, arrive late for activities and be
    inattentive and irritable.

14. *Learning to Satisfy Curiosity*
    Mental activity may be dulled.

## A METHOD TO ASSIST YOU IN ASSESSING MISS SCOTT'S DIFFICULTY

We would like to suggest you use the same sequence as before, that is:

● Complete the top half of the assessment sheet (*Figure 6.6*).
● Complete an individual profile of Miss Scott on re-occurrence of her
  symptoms, using as a guide sample profiles 7, 12, 14 in Chapter 2 Section 1.
● Complete the lower section of the assessment sheet.

We will leave you to devise her individual profile and would like you to
answer the following questions. Some suggestions for your answers will be at
the end of the chapter.

*Question 1.* Explain which of Miss Scott's physiological needs may be altered
in her present condition.

*Question 2.* Explain which of Miss Scott's security needs may be altered in
her present condition.

*Question 3.* Consider ways in which Miss Scott's achievement and self
fulfilment needs may be affected by her present state.

You can now check your completed assessment sheet with the one that follows
(*Figure 6.7*).

**Figure 6.6** *A patient profile to assist in assessing patients and the development of a problem-solving approach to care*

Name _____ Miss Scott _____ No. _____

Address _____

Circle any features that are present in your patient in each of the five columns. Remember that more than one is possible in most of the columns

Section A  1. Starting with the age column, take your selected condition and consider each of the 14 functions requiring assistance and tick in the box(es) those appropriate to your patient's needs, e.g. an elderly patient may require assistance with 2, 3 and 5

Section B  2. Repeat the same procedure with subsequent columns

**(A) Conditions always present that affect basic needs**

| | | | | Physiological disturbances |
|---|---|---|---|---|
| *Age* | *Temperament* | *Social/Cultural* | *Physical/Intellectual Capacity* | 1. Fluid and electrolyte imbalance |
| Newborn | Emotional state | Member of a family | | 2. Oxygen want |
| Child | or passing mode: | unit with friends | Normal weight | 3. Shock |
| Adolescent | (a) normal | and status | Over-weight | 4. Consciousness |
| Adult | (b) euphoric, | A person relatively | Under-weight | 5. Local injury/ disease |
| Middle aged | hyperactive | alone | Normal mentality | 6. Metabolism |
| Elderly | (c) anxious, fearful, | Maladjusted | Gifted mentality | 7. Seeing, hearing, smell and touch |
| Aged | agitated, | Destitute | Normal sense of: | 8. Communicable conditions |
| | hysterical | Smoker | hearing | 9. Immobilisation: disease/treatment |
| | (d) depressed/ | Drinker | sight | |
| | hypoactive | | equilibrium | |
| | | | touch | |
| | | | Loss of sense of: | |
| | | | hearing | |
| | | | sight | |
| | | | equilibrium | |
| | | | touch | |
| | | | Normal motor power | |
| | | | Loss of motor power | |

**(B)**

| Functions requiring assistance | *Age* | *Temperament* | *Social/Cultural* | *Physical/Intellectual Capacity* | *Physiological Disturbance* |
|---|---|---|---|---|---|
| 1. Breathing | | | | | |
| 2. Eating or drinking | | | | | |
| 3. Elimination | | | | | |
| 4. Sleep or rest | | | | | |
| 5. Movement | | | | | |
| 6. Maintenance of body temperature | | | | | |
| 7. Keeping body clean | | | | | |
| 8. Dressing suitably | | | | | |
| 9. Avoiding dangers and injury | | | | | |
| 10. Communication | | | | | |
| 11. Worship | | | | | |
| 12. Work | | | | | |
| 13. Participation in recreation | | | | | |
| 14. Learning to satisfy curiosity | | | | | |

**Figure 6.7**    *A patient profile to assist in assessing patients and the development of a problem-solving approach to care*

Name _____ Miss Scott _____ No. _____

Address _____

_____

Circle any features that are present in your patient in each of the five columns. Remember that more than one is possible in most of the columns

Section A    1. Starting with the age column, take your selected condition and consider each of the 14 functions requiring assistance and tick in the box(es) those appropriate to your patient's needs, e.g. an elderly patient may require assistance with 2, 3 and 5

Section B    2. Repeat the same procedure with subsequent columns

## Conditions always present that affect basic needs

### Physiological disturbances

**Age**
Newborn
Child
Adolescent
Adult
(Middle aged)
Elderly
Aged

**Temperament**
Emotional state or passing mode:
(a) normal
(b) euphoric, hyperactive
(c) (anxious, fearful,) agitated, hysterical
(d) depressed/ hypoactive

**Social/Cultural**
Member of a family unit with friends and status
(A person relatively alone)
Maladjusted
Destitute
Smoker
Drinker

**Physical/Intellectual Capacity**
Normal weight
Over-weight
(Under-weight)
(Normal mentality)
Gifted mentality
Normal sense of:
  hearing
  sight
  equilibrium
  touch
Loss of sense of:
  hearing
  sight
  equilibrium
  touch
(Normal motor power)
Loss of motor power

1. Fluid and electrolyte imbalance
2. Oxygen want
3. Shock
4. Consciousness
5. Local injury/ disease
6. (Metabolism)
7. Seeing, hearing, smell and touch
8. Communicable conditions
9. Immobilisation: disease/treatment

| Functions requiring assistance | Age | Temperament | Social/Cultural | Physical/Intellectual Capacity | Physiological Disturbance |
|---|---|---|---|---|---|
| 1. Breathing | | | | | ✓ |
| 2. Eating or drinking | | ✓ | | | ✓ |
| 3. Elimination | | ✓ | | | ✓ |
| 4. Sleep or rest | | ✓ | | | ✓ |
| 5. Movement | | ✓ | | | ✓ |
| 6. Maintenance of body temperature | | | | | ✓ |
| 7. Keeping body clean | | ✓ | | | ✓ |
| 8. Dressing suitably | | ✓ | | | ✓ |
| 9. Avoiding dangers and injury | | ✓ | | | ✓ |
| 10. Communication | | ✓ | | | ✓ |
| 11. Worship | | ✓ | | | ✓ |
| 12. Work | | ✓ | | | ✓ |
| 13. Participation in recreation | | ✓ | | | ✓ |
| 14. Learning to satisfy curiosity | | ✓ | | | ✓ |

You can now see that Miss Scott's temperament and disease process are the two factors influencing functions that are requiring assistance in order to enable her to meet her physiological, security, achievement and self-fulfilment needs.

## SELECTING NURSING ACTIONS TO ASSIST A PATIENT WITH DIFFICULTY IN SLEEPING AND RESTING

The main problem being discussed in this chapter is difficulty in sleeping and resting. We would now like you to choose from the following list of Nursing Actions those appropriate for Miss Scott by putting a tick in the appropriate column. Remember, ticking the Yes column helps you to decide on direct care and ticking the Maybe column indicates potential care that may be needed.

Whatever your decision, give an explanation of your choices and when you have completed this compare your decisions and explanations with those given on pages 174 to 175.

Table 6.2   *Nursing action to assist a patient with difficulty in sleeping and resting*

| Nursing actions | Yes | No | Maybe | Reason for choice |
|---|---|---|---|---|
| **Part 1   Breathing** | | | | |
| 1. Provide extra pillows | | | | |
| **Part 2   Eating and Drinking** | | | | |
| 1. Assist in completing menu requests | | | | |
| 2. Remind about mealtimes | | | | |
| 3. Provide meals | | | | |
| 4. Expect patient to carry on selecting, providing food as normal | | | | |
| 5. Encourage patient to eat and drink | | | | |
| 6. Cut up food and assist patient to eat | | | | |
| **Part 3   Eliminating** | | | | |
| 1. Give suppositories | | | | |
| 2. Give an aperient | | | | |
| **Part 4   Sleeping and Resting** | | | | |
| 1. Offer a warm drink on settling at night | | | | |
| 2. Give prescribed night sedation | | | | |
| 3. Position patient's bed in a quiet area of the ward | | | | |
| 4. Avoid making a noise near patient's bedside | | | | |

*Table 6.2   Continued*

| Nursing actions | Yes | No | Maybe | Reason for choice |
|---|---|---|---|---|
| **Part 4   Sleeping and Resting (continued)** | | | | |
| 5. Minimise use of lights at night | | | | |
| 6. Make sure the ward is bright enough for patient to see nurses | | | | |
| 7. Avoid unnecessary touching of patient and his or her bed at night | | | | |
| 8. Use a torch on patient's face to check patient is asleep and resting | | | | |
| 9. Place patient's bed near someone who is known to be a poor sleeper | | | | |
| **Part 5   Moving** | | | | |
| 1. Provide opportunity for patient to rest during the day | | | | |
| 2. Encourage constant activity during the day | | | | |
| 3. Keep patient at complete rest | | | | |
| 4. Encourage exercise | | | | |
| 5. Provide a sheepskin | | | | |
| 6. Provide a hoist | | | | |
| **Part 6   Maintaining Body Temperature** | | | | |
| 1. Provide light bedclothes | | | | |
| 2. Provide a fan | | | | |
| **Part 7   Keeping Body Clean** | | | | |
| 1. Give a daily bath on rising | | | | |
| 2. Assist patient washing in bed | | | | |
| 3. Encourage patient to bath before retiring | | | | |
| **Part 8   Dressing Suitably** | | | | |
| 1. Assist patient in choosing appropriate night clothes | | | | |
| **Part 9   Avoiding Danger and Injury** | | | | |
| 1. Alert patient to potential hazards in environment | | | | |
| 2. Check the environment is safe when patient settles and during the night | | | | |

*Table 6.2  Continued*

| Nursing actions | Yes | No | Maybe | Reason for choice |
|---|---|---|---|---|
| **Part 10  Communicating** | | | | |
| 1. Provide a call bell | | | | |
| 2. Be prepared to listen when patient is disturbed | | | | |
| 3. Discover reasons for waking | | | | |
| 4. Discourage patient from talking during the night | | | | |
| 5. Be discreet about confidences shared but report anything that is significant | | | | |
| 6. Respond promptly whenever patient has a query | | | | |
| 7. Discover patient's usual sleep pattern and practices | | | | |
| **Part 11  Worshipping** | | | | |
| 1. Ignore spiritual needs until the patient is feeling better | | | | |
| 2. Inform the night sister if patient requests to see the chaplain | | | | |
| **Part 12  Working** | | | | |
| 1. Report to day sister work-related problems | | | | |
| 2. Show an interest if and when patient wishes to talk about her work | | | | |
| 3. Discourage patient from talking about her work | | | | |
| **Part 13  Participating in Recreation** | | | | |
| 1. Allowed to read during the night if she wishes | | | | |
| 2. Allowed to use the hospital radio headphones during the night if she wishes | | | | |
| 3. Allowed to knit during the night if patient wishes | | | | |
| 4. All recreational activities to cease after 11 pm to ensure a good night's sleep | | | | |
| **Part 14  Learning to Satisfy Curiosity** | | | | |
| 1. Any question from the patient about her condition to be answered by the day staff | | | | |
| 2. Any queries from the patient to be answered as fully as possible | | | | |
| 3. Refer any questions not possible to answer during the night to day staff | | | | |

## EXPLANATION FOR CHOICE OF NURSING ACTIONS

### Part 1   Breathing

This should have been ticked in the Maybe column as she may be more comfortable sleeping with extra pillows.

### Part 2   Eating and Drinking

You should have ticked the Yes column for numbers 1, 2, 3 and 5, remembering that if someone has disturbed sleep she may not wish to bother with eating and drinking due to tiredness, and therefore encouragement will be required. You should have ticked the No column for numbers 4 and 6 as neither is appropriate.

### Part 3   Eliminating

You should have ticked the Maybe column for numbers 1 and 2 as these may be required as normal routine will have been disturbed.

### Part 4   Sleeping and Resting

You should have ticked in the Yes column numbers 1, 3, 4, 5 and 7 as all these measures promote comfort and reduce unnecessary stimuli from sounds, sights and touch. You should have ticked numbers 2 and 6 in the Maybe column as night sedation may have to be given since she is in a strange environment. For some patients being able to see what is happening at night can help reduce anxiety about what may be happening and the unknown. You should have ticked the No column for numbers 8 and 9 because a patient with sleeping difficulties will respond immediately to a torch light and to a nearby patient's demands.

### Part 5   Moving

You should have ticked the Yes column for number 1. If the patient has difficulty in sleeping at night extra rest may be required during the day. You should have ticked in the Maybe column numbers 4 and 5. Some exercise is necessary to maintain muscular movement, joint activity and the general circulation of the blood. A sheepskin may be necessary if the patient is particularly thin. The No column should have been ticked for numbers 2, 3 and 6. Numbers 2 and 3 are for the above reasons. A hoist is not likely to be needed for this active person.

### Part 6   Maintaining Body Temperature

You should have ticked the Yes column for number 1 as this patient might be restless. A fan may be necessary for the patient if she becomes hot and uncomfortable.

### Part 7   Keeping the Body Clean

You should have ticked the Yes column for number 3. She may need encouragement if feeling tired and a bath at night can be relaxing and promote sleep. The Maybe column should have been used for number 1. A bath on rising may be comforting if the patient has had a disturbed night. Number 2 should have been ticked in the No column as this would be inappropriate for this active patient.

**Part 8 Dressing Suitably**

You should have ticked this item in the Yes column as this patient may need advice on choosing light, loose and non-restrictive clothing.

*Part 9 Avoiding Danger and Injury*

You should have ticked the Yes column for both items as the patient may be too weary and be tempted to get up and wander around in her disturbed night.

*Part 10 Communicating*

You should have ticked the Yes column for numbers 1, 2, 3, 5, 6 and 7. A call bell can be useful and gives the patient confidence that she can attract attention during the night. Worries appear to be exaggerated at night and if the patient wishes to talk about them a nurse needs to respond by listening and showing an interest.

A nurse needs to consider other verbal and non-verbal cues given by the patient and attempt to discover usual sleep pattern, reasons for waking and other worries. Patients are often less inhibited during the night and may reveal confidences to a night nurse. The No column should have been used for number 4 as no opportunity should be lost for establishing contact and maintaining relationships with a patient.

*Part 11 Worshipping*

You should have ticked number 2 in the Yes column and number 1 in the No column as spiritual needs should be met promptly.

*Part 12 Working*

You should have ticked the Yes column for numbers 1 and 2 as this patient is in full-time employment and therefore work interests include a large part of her life and could give her financial worries due to losing work. Number 3 should have been used for the No column as this would be a hindrance for developing communication links with the patient.

*Part 13 Participating in Recreation*

You should have ticked the Yes column for numbers 1, 2 and 3 and the No column for number 4. It is more appropriate to allow the patient to relax with familiar activities rather than become frustrated lying awake in the dark.

*Part 14 Learning to Satisfy Curiosity*

You should have ticked the Yes column for numbers 2 and 3 and the No column for number 1. Night staff are part of the 24-hour nursing team and need to accept responsibility for sharing information with the patient.

You can now see that some of these Nursing Actions are dependent on the individual characteristics of Miss Scott and therefore her care plan needs to be sensitive to her individual needs. As we have suggested before you may like to discuss some of the suggested answers with your colleagues and/ or your tutor, as this will help you to question Nursing Actions.

Using *Table 6.3* we now ask you to identify priorities for planning the care that Miss Scott requires to help her with her difficulty in sleeping and resting.

## CHOOSING PRIORITIES IN NURSING ACTIONS

*Table 6.3   Priorities in nursing actions*

| Part | Insert your choice of priority numbers 1–14 |
|---|---|
| 1. Breathing | |
| 2. Eating and drinking | |
| 3. Eliminating | |
| 4. Sleeping and resting | |
| 5. Moving | |
| 6. Maintaining body temperature | |
| 7. Keeping body clean | |
| 8. Dressing suitably | |
| 9. Avoiding danger and injury | |
| 10. Communicating | |
| 11. Worshipping | |
| 12. Working | |
| 13. Participating in recreation | |
| 14. Learning to satisfy curiosity | |

You can now check your decision regarding priority choice of nursing actions with the plan given in *Table 6.4*.

If you wish to remind yourself about planning and providing nursing care please refer again to *Figure 3.4*, Section 2, Chapter 3.

## IDENTIFICATION OF CRITERIA FOR PROGRESS

You should now read carefully the plan shown in *Table 6.4* for identifying criteria for progress.

*Table 6.4   Plan of care for progress*

| Nursing actions to assist a patient with difficulty in sleeping and resting | Yes | Maybe | Priority Choice | Measurements | Short-term goals | Review period | Evaluation Criteria Have short-term goals been met? |
|---|---|---|---|---|---|---|---|
| **Part 4   Sleeping and Resting** | | | | Record:<br>(a) Length of sleep and number of disturbances during the night | 6–7 hours undisturbed sleep or rest | 24-hourly | Disturbed by noisy patient and emergency admission during night |
| 1. Offer a warm drink on settling at night | ✓ | | | | | | |
| 2. Give prescribed night sedation | | ✓ | | (b) If disturbed what has woken her | | | Woken each time sleeping pulse was taken |
| 3. Position patient's bed in a quiet area of the ward | ✓ | | | (c) Whether she wakes refreshed | | | Up early though still tired |
| 4. Avoid making a noise near patient's bedside | ✓ | | FIRST | (d) Whether night sedation is required | | | |
| 5. Minimise use of lights at night | ✓ | | | | | | |
| 6. Make sure the ward is bright enough for patient to see the nurses | | ✓ | | | | | |
| 7. Avoid unnecessary touching of patient and his or her bed at night | ✓ | | | | | | |
| **Part 10 Communicating** | | | | Note:<br>What worries are expressed and report as appropriate to day staff or night sister | Miss Scott is able to communicate and relate to staff caring for her at night | Ongoing | Seems fully aware of implications of treatment and length of stay in hospital. Miss Scott is exhibiting the expected response to her present condition, i.e. concern but not over anxious |
| 1. Provide a call bell | ✓ | | | | | | |
| 2. Be prepared to listen when patient is disturbed | ✓ | | | Whether explanations given are accepted | | | |
| 3. Discover reasons for waking | ✓ | | | Whether patient is excessively demanding, irritable or uncommunicative | | | |
| 5. Be discreet about confidences shared but report anything that is significant | ✓ | | SECOND | | | | |
| 6. Respond promptly whenever patient has a query | ✓ | | | | | | |
| 7. Discover patient's usual sleep pattern and practices | ✓ | | | | | | |
| **Part 14   Learning to Satisfy Curiosity** | | | | | | | |
| 2. To answer any queries from the patient as fully as possible | ✓ | | | | | | |

*Table 6.4    Continued*

| Nursing actions to assist a patient with difficulty in sleeping and resting | Yes | Maybe | Priority Choice | Measurements | Short-term goals | Review period | Evaluation Criteria Have short-term goals been met? |
|---|---|---|---|---|---|---|---|
| **Part 14   Learning to Satisfy Curiosity (continued)** | | | SECOND | | | | |
| 3. To refer any questions not possible to answer during the night to day sister | ✓ | | | | | | |
| **Part 11   Worshipping** | | | THIRD | Note the desire for spiritual help and assistance with work-related problems | Satisfaction of spiritual needs if necessary | 24-hourly | Links with own church maintained and likes to attend hospital chapel services |
| 2. Inform the night sister if patient requests to see the chaplain | ✓ | | | | Resolution of any outstanding work-related difficulties | | Has notified personnel department at her place of work |
| **Part 12   Working** | | | | | | | |
| 1. Report to day sister work-related problems | ✓ | | | | | | |
| 2. Show an interest if and when patient wishes to talk about her work | ✓ | | | | | | |
| **Part 5   Moving** | | | FOURTH | Note: Amount of activity during the night | Reduce the amount and frequency of activity to a minimal possible level | | When disturbed during the night patient went for a short walk, read a little and then resumed sleep |
| 1. Provide opportunity for patient to rest during the day | ✓ | | | Nature of activity during the night | Ensure there is a safe environment | | |
| 4. Encourage exercise | | ✓ | | Record and report any hazards in the ward area | | | |
| 5. Provide a sheepskin | | ✓ | | | | | |
| **Part 9   Avoiding Danger and Injury** | | | | | | | |
| 1. Alert patient to potential hazards in environment | ✓ | | | | | | |
| 2. Check the environment is safe when patient settles and during the night | ✓ | | | | | | |
| **Part 13   Participating in Recreation** | | | | | | | |
| 1. Allowed to read during the night if she wishes | ✓ | | | | | | |
| 2. Allowed to use hospital radio headphones during the night if she wishes | ✓ | | | | | | |

*Table 6.4 Continued*

| Nursing actions to assist a patient with difficulty in sleeping and resting. | Yes | Maybe | Priority Choice | Measurements | Short-term goals | Review period | Evaluation Criteria Have short-term goals been met? |
|---|---|---|---|---|---|---|---|
| **Part 13 Participating in Recreation (continued)**<br><br>3. Allowed to knit during the night if patient wishes | ✓ | | FOURTH | Record body temperature on settling to sleep | Body temperature maintained within normal limits | 24-hourly | No rise in temperature recorded and feels comfortable |
| **Part 6 Maintaining Body Temperature**<br><br>1. Provide light bedclothes | ✓ | | FIFTH | | | | |
| 2. Provide a fan | | ✓ | | | | | |
| **Part 8 Dressing Suitably**<br><br>1. Assist patient in choosing appropriate night clothes | ✓ | | | | | | |
| **Part 2 Eating and Drinking**<br><br>1. Assist in completing menu requests | ✓ | | SIXTH | Record fluid intake and output if these are of concern<br><br>Note any hunger or thirst during the night and difficulty with elimination | Hydration and nutrition is maintained with satisfactory elimination | 12-hourly (a.m.) | Appreciates cup of tea when awakened<br><br>Doesn't appear to be hungry<br><br>Doesn't appear to have any difficulties with elimination |
| 2. Remind about mealtimes | ✓ | | | | | | |
| 4. Provide meals | ✓ | | | | | | |
| 5. Encourage patient to eat and drink | ✓ | | | | | | |
| **Part 3 Eliminating**<br><br>1. Give suppositories | | ✓ | | | | | |
| 2. Give an aperient | | ✓ | | | | | |
| **Part 7 Keeping the Body Clean**<br><br>1. Give a daily bath on rising | | ✓ | SEVENTH | Note her ability to attend to her own hygiene | Fully able to care for her own hygiene | 24-hourly | Enjoys having a bath before going to bed |
| 3. Encourage patient to bath before retiring | ✓ | | | | | | |
| **Part 1 Breathing**<br><br>1. Provide extra pillows | | ✓ | EIGHTH | Note any difficulty in breathing | Able to breathe normally | 24-hourly | No problems experienced |

### Using Evaluation Criteria for Resetting Short-term Goals

We would like to suggest that you reconsider Miss Scott's evaluation criteria after the first 24 hours in hospital and decide on new priorities for nursing action, revised measurements and setting of new short-term goals for preparing her for surgery (partial thyroidectomy).

## CONCLUSION

If you are going to look after this patient you will need to consider how her condition affects other living difficulties and you may like to discuss this as a further exercise. In this patient history we are not in a position to identify the long-term goals of Miss Scott. However these will be directed towards her resuming her usual living activities and satisfying her own needs. This chapter, we hope, will assist you in planning the care of other patients who have difficulty in sleeping and resting due to other conditions.

## CONDITIONS WHICH AFFECT SLEEPING AND RESTING

People can have difficulty in sleeping and resting without necessarily having a medical or a surgical condition, so we have included a brief discussion of insomnia and disturbance of biorhythms due to shift working or travel. As well as an illness or condition that affects sleeping and resting we have included at the end of the chapter some references to other conditions that cause coma or unconsciousness.

### Insomnia

Insomnia is sleeplessness. Most commonly associated with worry, this very common type of sleeplessness is always about something real or relevant, e.g. night before moving home, before an important interview, examination(s) or an operation. There is often no solution to them but you continue to worry about them. The bed which is normally inviting, warm or cosy no longer seems a friendly place and contains bumps or hollows never noticed before and you change position time and time again. You are easily distracted by normally familiar sounds and lights. Insomnia related to this type of worry resolves as soon as the event passes.

### Long-term Worry

This can lead to chronic insomnia which is more complicated. Again there may be a worry about real problems such as illness, work or money or having too much responsibility. These problems are unlikely to be resolved in a few days and the worries return night after night and frequently during the day as well. When the problem causing the worry improves, the insomnia improves but once the pattern of sleeplessness becomes established it will not alter. There are other worries about real problems which are not so easily resolved. Thoughts and doubts about death and the after life, the meaning of life and being and the power of the supernatural can return again and again. These are problems which are of concern to us all but for some they demand an answer even though the mind is incapable of giving one and sleeplessness is the result. In the severest form these ideas are called obsessional ruminations.

### Insomnia Due to 'Imaginary Fears'

During the night, however, these fears are real enough but in fact they are fears about things which should not make us afraid. These may include fears about physical health, losing consciousness and control and of dying in the night, in the absence of physical illness. These fears can be the key features of hypochondriasis. The hypochrondriac lying in bed at night is all too conscious of his bodily functions: he hears his breathing, is aware of the heart beating, feels his stomach rumbling, his ears popping, joints twingeing and muscles contracting. Any unexpected change such as his heart missing a beat is liable to set in motion a chain of worry.

### Sleep Rhythms

The normal activity in Britain is night sleep, day work, evening play, night sleep. This mirrors our normal body rhythms with their characteristic lower level at night and higher level during the day. Body rhythms come in many lengths. We are most concerned here with daily or Circadian rhythms which are characterised by a twenty-four hour oscillation with a night low, and a day high. In the absence of all environmental time cues, body rhythms run free at their individual day lengths, but in the real world environmental time cues lock all Circadian rhythms into the common twenty-four hour day length bringing them into harmony with each other. The regular change from light to dark is the most powerful cue for animals and plants but for human beings social cues are even stronger.

### Travellers and Shift Workers

Work, play, sleep sequence are out of harmony with body time. For example, for night workers when body clocks signal a low the night worker must be alert and when the body clock signals a high the night worker tries to sleep. Similarly when a traveller travels westward he may take off from London in the morning and arrive in New York at an earlier time in the same morning even though the flight has taken several hours. He gets out of the aircraft after a full day's travelling but instead of taking a well-earned sleep he has to face another day. It is commonly thought that the individual's body rhythms are reset over several days to adjust to the new routine, but later studies have shown that this is probably not so. See Smith and Wedderburn (1980).

### Change of Environment and/or Routine

Insomnia caused by much smaller changes in sleep pattern is very common. People may insist they cannot sleep properly away from the security and comfort of their own bedroom. They retire to bed the same time each night and are very fussy about the night clothes they wear, the temperature of the bedroom, the colour and texture of the sheets and the number of blankets. Such things need to be borne in mind when patients are admitted into the strange environment and routine of a hospital ward.

## REFERENCES, FURTHER READING AND TECHNIQUES

### References

Green, J. H. (1978). *Basic Clinical Physiology*, 3rd edition. Oxford University Press, Oxford.

Hunt, P and Sendell, B. (1987). *Nursing the Adult with a Specific Physiological Disturbance*. Macmillan Education, London.

Smith, P. and Wedderburn, Z. (1980). Sleep, body rhythms and shift work, *Nursing (Oxford)*, **20**, pages 889–892.

### Suggested Further Reading

*Related to Medical Conditions Affecting Sleeping and Resting*
Macleod, J. (Ed.). *Davidson's Principles and Practice of Medicine*, 13th edition. Churchill Livingstone, Edinburgh, 1983: Chapter 3 pp. 49–71; Chapter 11 pp. 458–533; Chapter 14 pp. 649–727; Chapter 15 pp. 755–780.
Read, A. E., Barritt, D. W. and Hewer, R. *Modern Medicine*, 3rd edition. Pitman Medical, London, 1984: Chapter 2 pp. 13–27; Chapter 12 pp. 194–226; Chapter 21 pp. 472–532; Chapter 22 pp. 533–619.

These books include:
● Infectious diseases
● Conditions of the nervous system
● Mental health
● Metabolic and endocrine disturbances

*Related to Surgical Conditions Affecting Sleeping and Resting*
Collins, S. and Parker, E. (Ed.). *Introduction to Nursing*. Essentials of Nursing Series, Macmillan, London, 1987.
Ellis, H. and Wastell, C. *General Surgery for Nurses*. Blackwell Scientific, Oxford, Chapter 16 pp. 369–381.
Henderson, M. A. *Essential Surgery for Nurses*. Churchill Livingstone, 1980, Chapter 15 pp. 58–61.
Horton, R. *General Surgery and the Nurse*. Hodder and Stoughton, London 1983, Chapter 9 pp. 57–68.

These books include:
● Thyroid disease
● Thyroidectomy
● Pain management

### Pharmacology Related to Care of Patients with Difficulty in Sleeping and Resting

You may wish to familiarize yourself with the medicines commonly used for patients with difficulty in sleeping and resting.
● Hypnotics
● Narcotics
● Sedatives
● Analgesics
See Jestico, J. V. (1980). Night sedation and sleep, *Nursing (Oxford)*, **20** pages 886–888.

### Suggested Nursing Procedures / Guidelines for Nursing Practice

You may wish to familiarise yourself with your local policies and procedures for administration of medicines or any other procedures which may be applicable to a patient requiring assistance with difficulty in sleeping and resting.

### SUGGESTED ANSWERS REGARDING INDIVIDUAL PROFILE OF MISS SCOTT

*Question 1.* Miss Scott's need for food and drink, elimination, exercise, rest and sleep are altering during her present state; refer to Effects of Difficulty in Sleeping and Resting on Living Activities (pages 167–168).

*Question 2*. For safety at home and work refer to page 168 as for Question 1, particularly numbers 9 and 12. For sense of belonging refer to number 13 Participating in Recreation.

*Question 3*. All of the needs in these two sections may be affected due to lack of drive and energy.

## Chapter 7

# Multiple Living Activities

## INTRODUCTION

Up to this point we have taken one living activity for detailed examination in
each chapter, covering Breathing, Eating and Drinking, Eliminating and
Sleeping and Resting. It is now time to consider a patient who may have all her
living activities affected by her present state of health, temperament, social
setting and mental and physical capabilities.

We now ask you to study how the remaining living activities, i.e. Moving,
Maintenance of body temperature, Keeping body clean, Dressing suitably,
Avoiding injury and danger, Communicating, Worshipping, Working, Participating in recreation and Learning and satisfying curiosity, are affected by
sociological and psychological factors and pathological states. Each of the
remaining living activities and some of the factors which affect them are
presented as a series of information sheets (Figures *7.1* to *7.10*). These are by
no means exhaustive and you may wish to add more, derived from your own
experience.

The chapter continues with a patient history from which we will be asking
you to assess, plan and evaluate care and the patient's progress. By bringing all
these factors together in considering one individual patient we hope you can
see how a personalised approach can be undertaken no matter how many living
activities are affected. Suggested further reading is given at end of the chapter.

## NORMAL PHYSIOLOGY

Before proceeding we suggest you revise your knowledge of normal physiology
related to Moving, Maintenance of body temperature, Keeping body clean,
Dressing suitably, Avoiding injuries and danger and Communicating by using
the following references or any other suitable textbook.

- Hunt and Sendell (1987). *Nursing the Adult with a Specific Physiological
  Disturbance*.
  Nervous system.
  Skeletal and muscular system.
  Defence systems of the body.
  Body defences against injury and disease.
  Special senses.
  Maintenance of blood pressure and circulation.
- Green (1978). *Basic Clinical Physiology*, pages 153–163.

**Figure 7.1**   *Factors affecting moving*

Moving is normally independent, active, enabling avoidance of dangers, assisting in a sense of well-being and can be a form of artistic expression.

**Sociological factors**
Participating in sports
Relaxation: yoga
Economic:
   walking
   public transport
   private transport
Maintenance and legislation regarding
vehicles
Access to buildings for the elderly/disabled
Others.................................................
   .............................................
   .............................................

**Psychological factors**
Gestures
Non-verbal communication
Use of body language
Use of personal space
   sexual partnerships
   interpersonal relationships
Others ...............................................
   .............................................
   .............................................

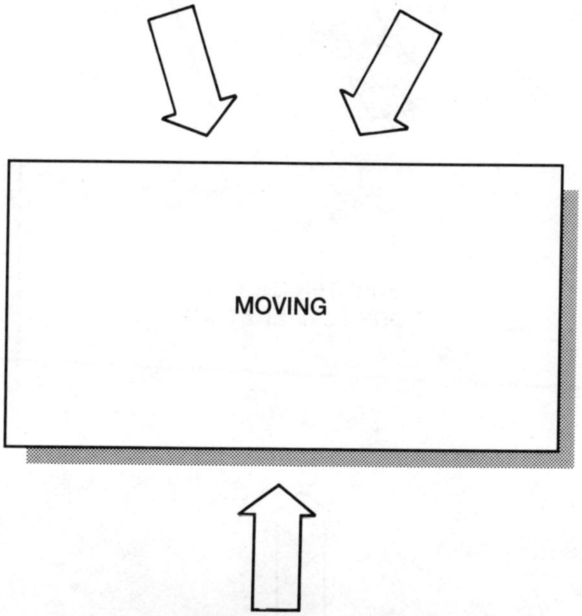

**MOVING**

**Pathological states**
Congenital, e.g. spastic paralysis
Injuries, e.g. fractures
Disease, e.g.
   cerebrovascular accidents
   multiple sclerosis
   nervous ticks/twitches
   catatonic states
   epilepsy

Others ...............................................
   .............................................
   .............................................

**Figure 7.2**    *Factors affecting maintenance of body temperature*

Allows optimum temperature range for enzyme and hormone activity.

**Sociological factors**
Provision of adequate shelter
Heating of homes
Conventions of dress and clothing
Adequate nutrition
Ventilation of homes and work places

Others ..................................................................

.............................................................

.............................................................

**Psychological factors**
Promotes a sense of well-being and
encourages and stimulates
activity both mental and
physical

Others ..................................................................

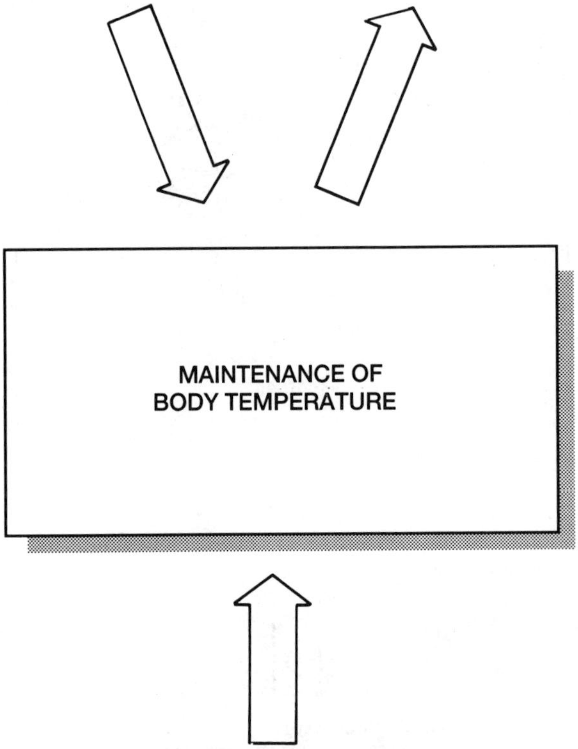

..................................................................

..................................................................

**MAINTENANCE OF
BODY TEMPERATURE**

**Pathological states**
Infection: hyperpyrexia, fever, rigor
Exposure: hypothermia (cold)/hyperpyrexia
(excessive heat)
Disease: myxoedema
Injuries: head injuries affecting temperature
control centre

Others ..................................................................

.............................................................

.............................................................

**Figure 7.3**  *Factors affecting keeping the body clean*

A frequent activity which can indicate a state of social, psychological and physical well-being.

**Sociological factors**
Availability of water, e.g.
  in developing areas
  droughts
  floods
Provision of water supply to:
  communal points
  individual houses
Nomads may use alternatives, e.g. mud/ochre
Vagrants use public facilities
Provision of baths/showers

Others ...............................................
  ...............................................
  ...............................................

**Psychological factors**
Morale booster:
  feel better
  look better
Remove odours: use of perfumes/deodorants
Ritual cleansing:
  before ceremonies
  before meals
  before religious practices

Others ...............................................
  ...............................................
  ...............................................

KEEPING THE BODY CLEAN

**Pathological states**
Infestations
Skin diseases
Depression
Any debilitating illness

Others ...............................................
  ...............................................
  ...............................................

**Figure 7.4**   *Factors affecting dressing suitably*

Establishes identity and independence as an individual and as a member of a group. Protects the individual from the environment and can be purely decorative.

**Sociological factors**
Cultural and group influences
Climate
Economic:
   utility
   status
Others ...............................................................
   ...............................................................
   ...............................................................

**Psychological factors**
Personal likes and dislikes
Morale booster
Conforming to group norms:
   mods
   T-shirts/jeans
   punks
   school uniform
   uniform at work
Use of dress for self-expression

Others ...............................................................
   ...............................................................
   ...............................................................

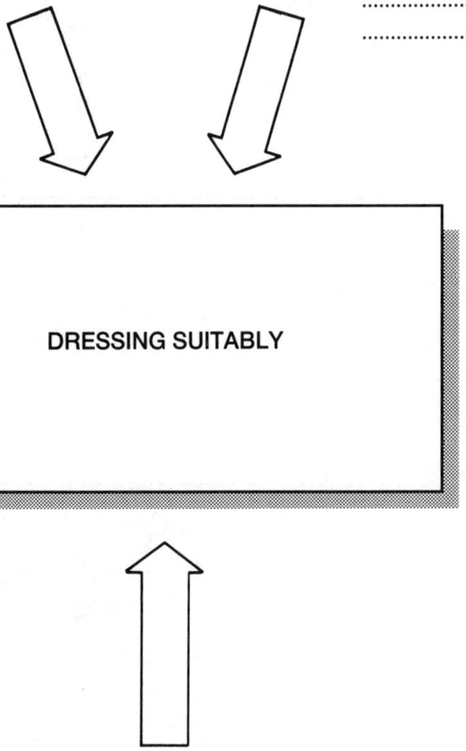

**DRESSING SUITABLY**

**Pathological states**
Helpless, disabled, incontinent due to
   a congenital or degenerative physical or
   mental disease or condition
Injuries causing disability

Others ...............................................................
   ...............................................................
   ...............................................................

**Figure 7.5**  *Factors affecting avoidance of dangers and injury*

Necessary to respond to the environment in order to survive and maintain function as an individual.

**Sociological factors**
Health and Safety at Work Acts
Factory Acts
   clean air
   food
   protective clothing
   occupational health
   local policies and procedures
'At risk' registers for:
   babies
   elderly
Health Education:
   smoking
   sexually transmitted diseases
   pregnancy
   drugs (misuse of)
   chemical abuse, e.g. glue sniffing
Others ...............................................................
   ...............................................................
   ...............................................................

**Psychological factors**
Perception of danger
Learning avoidance of hazards
Self-preservation:
   individual
   group
   species
Vulnerable groups:
   children
   elderly
Others ...............................................................
   ...............................................................
   ...............................................................

**AVOIDING DANGERS AND INJURY**

**Pathological states**
Loss of sight, hearing, feeling
Phobias
Self-destruction—suicide
Hysterical response
Any disease/injury causing helplessness and
   inability to protect from danger
Others ...............................................................
   ...............................................................
   ...............................................................

**Figure 7.6**   *Factors affecting communicating*

A two-way process of social interaction, and is dependent on the person's ability to speak and interpret appropriate language and to use and recognise non-verbal gestures, expressions and body language.

**Sociological factors**
Use of familiar and unfamiliar languages,
   dialects and abbreviations
Rituals and customs:
  ceremonials
  dancing
  speech making
'Official' language:
  law
  technology
Use of media:
  TV
  Advertising
  Newspapers
  Books
Others .....................................................
    .....................................................
    .....................................................

**Psychological factors**
Perception
Learning:
  literacy
  numeracy
Intelligence quotient
Propaganda—use of media
Development of interpersonal skills

Others ...............................................................
   .................................................................
   .................................................................

### COMMUNICATING

**Pathological states**
Loss or defect of sight, hearing, speech,
Defects in:
  personality development
  learning (dyslexia and literacy)
Injury/disease of central nervous system

Others ................................................................
   ..............................................................
   ..............................................................

**Figure 7.7**   *Factors affecting worshipping*

Some form of worshipping is adopted by most societies in the world and can be individual or formalised in the rituals and practices of the world religions.

**Sociological factors**
The practices and rituals of the main religions can affect, e.g.
   behaviour
   choice of food
   choice of dress
The 'Work Ethic'
   provides a caring community
   outside the family
Others .................................................
   .................................................
   .................................................

**Psychological factors**
Need for belief in 'after life'
Psychological 'prop'
Promotes interaction
Identifies:
   moral dilemmas
   ethical dilemmas
Others .................................................
   .................................................
   .................................................

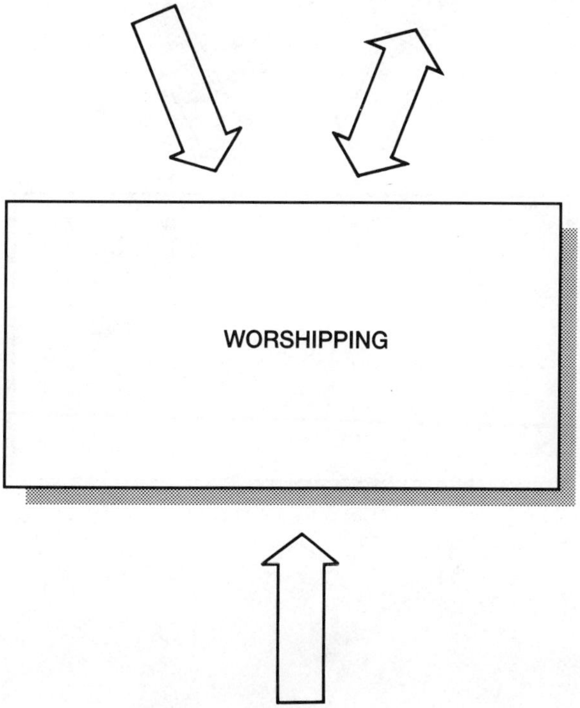

## WORSHIPPING

**Pathological states**
Mental illnesses:
   delusions
   mania
Any disease/injury which prevents
communal worshipping
Others .................................................
   .................................................
   .................................................

**Figure 7.8** *Factors affecting working*

Promotes a sense of achievement, self-fulfilment and provides an economic means of providing for self and others. Provides a reason for mental and physical activity.

**Sociological factors**
Provides an income
Enables support of others
Enables share of rewards, e.g.
   giving to charities
   exchanging gifts
Extends social contacts
Provides merchandise/expertise for:
   trade and industry
   essential community services

Others ..................................................
.........................................................
.........................................................

**Psychological factors**
Stimulates drive/motivation
Assists in gaining self-respect
  and confidence
Satisfies super-ego

Others ..................................................
.........................................................
.........................................................

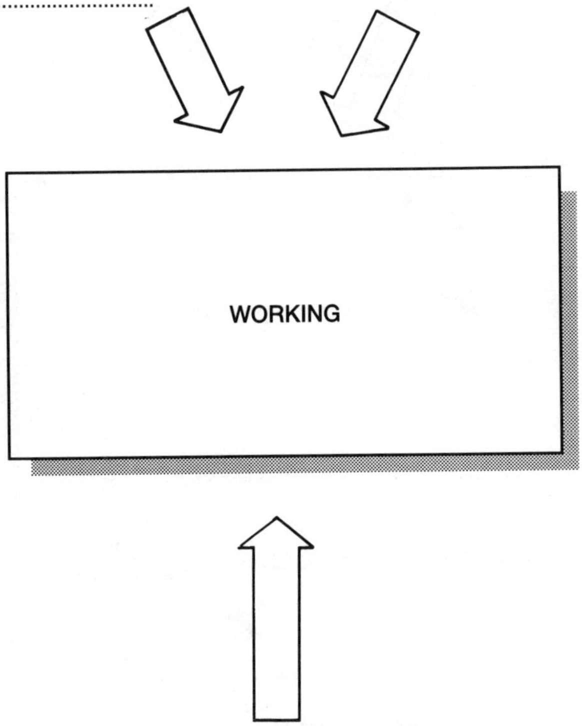

**WORKING**

**Pathological states**
Any disease or condition which
  prevents working
Interruption to working due to injury

Others ..................................................
.........................................................
.........................................................

**Figure 7.9**  *Factors affecting participation in recreation*

Provides mental and physical stimulation and assists in preventing illness and promoting well-being.

**Sociological factors**
Recreation is dependent on what is currently
    fashionable/being promoted
Provides an alternative activity to employment
Can be creative and possibly productive
Promotes group/national/international image
Others ...............................................................
    ...............................................................
    ...............................................................

**Psychological factors**
Increases self-respect and self-confidence
Promotes sharing and group dynamics/support
Sense of purpose
Release of tension
Others ...............................................................
    ...............................................................
    ...............................................................

**PARTICIPATING IN RECREATION**

**Pathological states**
Any injury/disease or condition which affects
    mobility and/or concentration, e.g.
    nervous or locomotor diseases
    mental depression
Others ...............................................................
    ...............................................................
    ...............................................................

**Figure 7.10** *Factors affecting learning and satisfying curiosity*

A means of development of the individual and society. Gives a sense of security and being in control of a situation.

**Sociological factors**
Cultural 'norms'
Provision of educational facilities
Provision of research and expertise for
  development of knowledge
Communications:
  information
  technology
Others ...............................................................
      ...............................................................
      ...............................................................

**Psychological factors**
Learning theories:
  discovery
  trial and error
  experiential
Pavlov's dogs
Motivation:
  goal setting
  assessments
Emotions:
  hunger
  noise (can inhibit)

Others ...............................................................
      ...............................................................
      ...............................................................

LEARNING AND SATISFYING
CURIOSITY

**Pathological states**
Congenital defects—educationally subnormal
Disease or injury which can cause intellectual
  disablement

Others ...............................................................
      ...............................................................
      ...............................................................

## PATIENT HISTORY

We would now like you to consider a patient who has difficulty with all the living activities due to a cerebrovascular accident. See also Hunt and Sendell (1987).

Mrs Robinson, aged 72 years, lives with her 80-year-old husband and his sister, Mrs Edwards, a widow aged 78 years, in a large Victorian house in a neglected area of a major city. The upper part of the house is let as bed-sitters, occupied by two students. The house has a flight of six steps up to the front door and the only bathroom and toilet is on the first floor. There is a small garden at the rear but as the house is built on a hill there are several steps up to it. The nearest shops are at the bottom of a steep hill but on a bus route. The hospital is at the far side of the city centre. Mrs Robinson, the most active member of the family, does most of the shopping, cooking and housework although her sister-in-law has taken responsibility for the family's washing and ironing. Mr Robinson enjoys propagating seeds and cuttings in his small greenhouse but is no longer able to look after the heavy work in the garden.

After a morning's housework Mrs Robinson was found by her sister-in-law on the floor in the kitchen. Mrs Edwards was unable to rouse her and was frightened by Mrs Robinson's noisy breathing and odd colour. She called her brother and went next door to ask the neighbour to get help. They tried to make Mrs Robinson comfortable on the floor but were both very anxious by the time the doctor arrived. The doctor examined Mrs Robinson and, suspecting that she had suffered a cerebro-vascular accident, arranged for her immediate transfer to the medical ward of the local hospital.

On arrival the following observations are made:

- Deeply unconscious
- Limbs flaccid and reflexes absent
- Pupils equal but reacting sluggishly
- Breathing stertorous
- Colour pale and slightly cyanosed
- Swallowing and coughing reflexes absent
- Incontinent of urine
- Pulse 90 beats per minute
- Blood pressure 130/90 mmHg
- Temperature 36.8°C

### Explanation of Abnormal Physiology and Pathology

Any interruption of the blood supply to the brain *or* any injury to the nerve cells and/or nerve pathways within the brain *or* any increase of pressure within the cranium will result in loss of, or reduction in, the function of that part of the brain affected and the organs and tissues supplied by the affected nerves (see *Table 7.1*).

*Table 7.1   Normal and abnormal physiology*

| Normal physiology | Abnormal physiology |
|---|---|
| (a) Conscious state, aware of surroundings and responsive to stimuli, depends on healthy brain tissue and good blood supply | Sudden loss of consciousness due to haemorrhage from a cerebral artery which results in lack of blood to the area of brain tissue distal to the site of rupture of the vessel |
| (b) Central nervous system: motor nerves maintain muscle tone and activity | Pressure of leaking blood on motor pathways interrupts nerve impulses to the muscles on the opposite side of the body causing loss of muscle tone and flaccid paralysis |
| (c) Sensory nerve pathways bring information of pain, touch, temperature and pressure from the body to the brain | Pressure of leaking blood on the sensory pathways interrupts the impulses bringing information to the brain from the opposite side of the body |
| (d) Protective reflexes situated in the medulla oblongata operate below the level of consciousness to protect against, for example, inhalation of saliva or vomit | Pressure within the cranium rises due to the haemorrhage which compresses the medulla oblongata. This inhibits the swallowing and coughing reflexes. |
| (e) Vital centres such as respiratory, vasomotor and temperature-regulating function in conjunction with the autonomic nervous system | Damage to brain tissue or raised intracranial pressure compresses the nerve centres and inhibits activity causing difficulty in breathing, poor temperature control and changes in the blood pressure |
| (f) Oculomotor nerve (3rd cranial nerve) controls the size of the pupils to regulate the amount of light to the retina | Damage or pressure on the oculomotor nerve can cause sluggish reaction of the pupil to light or unequal pupil response to light |
| (g) Centres in the dominant hemisphere of the brain permit articulation of speech | Damage or pressure on the dominant hemisphere may result in dysphasia |

### Mrs Robinson's Recovery and Rehabilitation

Mrs Robinson remains deeply unconscious for five days and then starts to open her eyes. Some spontaneous movement of the left side of her body returns. The right hemiplegia becomes more obvious. She starts to suck anything put in her mouth and seems to be swallowing her saliva. Her eyes appear to focus but she makes no attempt to speak. She has a worried expression on her face and becomes agitated when approached. Having become aware of the nasogastric tube and urinary catheter, she attempts to remove both. Oral fluids are gradually reintroduced and when sufficient fluid is taken for daily requirements the nasogastric tube is removed. She experiences difficulty with dribbling due to paralysis of facial muscles. A rehabilitation programme is started, involving the nursing staff, physiotherapist, speech therapist and occupational therapist for preparation for return to daily living, that is: regaining balance in bed, in chair and standing; teaching to walk and manage stairs; visiting the toilet; eating and drinking at table; washing and dressing; developing ability to talk and communicate. The urinary catheter was removed when Mrs Robinson was able to use the sani-chair.

During this time the medical social worker and occupational therapist carry out a home assessment to determine the feasability of Mrs Robinson's returning home if left with residual hemiplegia or dysphasia. Joint discussion between nursing staff, medical, paramedical staff and relatives decide which support services will be required for transfer to the community.

It is advisable to revise the Bobath technique for the care of patients following cerebrovascular accident.

## EFFECTS OF MRS ROBINSON'S PRESENT STATE ON LIVING ACTIVITIES

### Multiple Difficulties

1. *Breathing*
   Now independent and quiet.

2. *Eating and Drinking*
   Nasogastric tube is now removed and she is beginning to swallow fluids but still dribbles due to paralysis of facial muscles.

3. *Eliminating*
   Still difficult due to paralysis. Needs help to walk to the lavatory or to use sani-chair.

4. *Sleeping and Resting*
   Gets tired easily, needs to rest during the day. Sleep disturbed due to inability to reposition herself in bed because of residual paralysis.

5. *Moving*
   Needs to relearn how to balance in bed, in a chair, and how to use utensils for eating and drinking. When standing she needs to be taught to walk and climb stairs, use toilet, and to wash and dress.

6. *Maintaining Body Temperature*
   Dependent on others to choose clothing and alter bedclothes according to the temperature of the environment.

7. *Keeping Body Clean*
   Dependent on others to teach her and assist her to care for her skin, hair, nails.

8. *Dressing Suitably*
   Dependent on others to teach and assist her to choose and dress suitably.

9. *Avoiding Dangers and Injuries*
   Dependent on others for identification and protection from environmental hazards.

10. *Communicating*
    Appears to see and hear but is having difficulty in speaking. Is dependent on others to spend time to assist her and teach her to communicate. Will require aids. Non-verbal cues may be misleading as her worried expression may be due to her facial paralysis.

11. *Worshipping*
    Further information may be needed regarding her spiritual needs.

12. *Working*
    She is going to be unable to do the shopping, cooking and housework at home.

13. *Participating in Recreation*
    Dependent on others to arrange this but it could be a useful stimulus to her rehabilitation.

14. *Learning and Satisfying Curiosity*
    As communication skills develop, she will be kept informed about her progress and participate in planning for her future.

**ASSESSMENT OF MRS ROBINSON**

We have shown you in previous chapters how to use profiles from Section 1 in deciding how a patient would normally satisfy basic needs and to super-impose the specific needs due to a pathological state on admission to hospital Would you now do this for Mrs Robinson using the assessment sheet (*Figure 7.11*) and check your ideas with the completed sheet that follows (*Figure 7.12*). You may find there are some discrepancies as we are dealing with a hypothetical situation.

**Figure 7.11** *A patient profile to assist in assessing patients and the development of a problem-solving approach to care*

---

Name **Mrs Robinson following**  No. _____

Address **cerebrovascular accident**

_____

Circle any features that are present in your patient in each of the five columns. Remember that more than one is possible in most of the columns

Section A  1. Starting with the age column, take your selected condition and consider each of the 14 functions requiring assistance and tick in the box(es) those appropriate to your patient's needs, e.g. an elderly patient may require assistance with 2, 3 and 5

Section B  2. Repeat the same procedure with subsequent columns

---

**(A) Conditions always present that affect basic needs**

| Age | Temperament | Social/Cultural | Physical/Intellectual Capacity | **Physiological disturbances** |
|---|---|---|---|---|
| Newborn | Emotional state | Member of a family | Normal weight | 1. Fluid and electrolyte imbalance |
| Child | or passing mode: | unit with friends | Over-weight | 2. Oxygen want |
| Adolescent | (a) normal | and status | Under-weight | 3. Shock |
| Adult | (b) euphoric, | A person relatively | Normal mentality | 4. Consciousness |
| Middle aged | hyperactive | alone | Gifted mentality | 5. Local injury/ disease |
| Elderly | (c) anxious, fearful, | Maladjusted | Normal sense of: | 6. Metabolism |
| Aged | agitated, | Destitute | hearing | 7. Seeing, hearing, smell and touch |
| | hysterical | Smoker | sight | 8. Communicable conditions |
| | (d) depressed/ | Drinker | equilibrium | 9. Immobilisation: disease/treatment |
| | hypoactive | | touch | |
| | | | Loss of sense of: | |
| | | | hearing | |
| | | | sight | |
| | | | equilibrium | |
| | | | touch | |
| | | | Normal motor power | |
| | | | Loss of motor power | |

---

**(B)**

| Functions requiring assistance | Age | Temperament | Social/Cultural | Physical/Intellectual Capacity | Physiological Disturbance |
|---|---|---|---|---|---|
| 1. Breathing | | | | | |
| 2. Eating or drinking | | | | | |
| 3. Elimination | | | | | |
| 4. Sleep or rest | | | | | |
| 5. Movement | | | | | |
| 6. Maintenance of body temperature | | | | | |
| 7. Keeping body clean | | | | | |
| 8. Dressing suitably | | | | | |
| 9. Avoiding dangers and injury | | | | | |
| 10. Communication | | | | | |
| 11. Worship | | | | | |
| 12. Work | | | | | |
| 13. Participation in recreation | | | | | |
| 14. Learning to satisfy curiosity | | | | | |

**Figure 7.12**   *A patient profile to assist in assessing patients and the development of a problem-solving approach to care*

---

Name   **Mrs Robinson following**   No. _____

Address   **cerebrovascular accident**

Section A   Circle any features that are present in your patient in each of the five columns. Remember that more than one is possible in most of the columns

Section B   1. Starting with the age column, take your selected condition and consider each of the 14 functions requiring assistance and tick in the box(es) those appropriate to your patient's needs, e.g. an elderly patient may require assistance with 2, 3 and 5

2. Repeat the same procedure with subsequent columns

**(A)   Conditions always present that affect basic needs**

**Physiological disturbances**

| Age | Temperament | Social/Cultural | Physical/Intellectual Capacity | Physiological disturbances |
|---|---|---|---|---|
| Newborn | Emotional state or passing mode: | Member of a family unit with friends and status | Capacity | 1. Fluid and electrolyte imbalance |
| Child | (a) normal | A person relatively alone | Normal weight | 2. Oxygen want |
| Adolescent | (b) euphoric, hyperactive | Maladjusted | Over-weight | 3. Shock |
| Adult | (c) anxious, fearful, agitated, hysterical | Destitute | Under-weight | 4. Consciousness |
| Middle aged | (d) depressed/ hypoactive | Smoker | Normal mentality | 5. Local injury/ disease |
| Elderly | | Drinker | Gifted mentality | 6. Metabolism |
| Aged | | | Normal sense of: hearing, sight, equilibrium, touch | 7. Seeing, hearing, smell and touch |
| | | | Loss of sense of: hearing, sight, equilibrium, touch | 8. Communicable conditions |
| | | | Normal motor power | 9. Immobilisation: disease/treatment |
| | | | Loss of motor power | |

**(B)**

| Functions requiring assistance | Age | Temperament | Social/Cultural | Physical/Intellectual Capacity | Physiological Disturbance |
|---|---|---|---|---|---|
| 1. Breathing | | | | | |
| 2. Eating or drinking | | | | ✓ | ✓ |
| 3. Elimination | | | | ✓ | ✓ |
| 4. Sleep or rest | | | | | ✓ |
| 5. Movement | | | | ✓ | ✓ |
| 6. Maintenance of body temperature | | | | | ✓ |
| 7. Keeping body clean | | | | ✓ | ✓ |
| 8. Dressing suitably | | | | ✓ | ✓ |
| 9. Avoiding dangers and injury | | | | ✓ | ✓ |
| 10. Communication | | ✓ | | ✓ | ✓ |
| 11. Worship | | | | | ✓ |
| 12. Work | | | | ✓ | ✓ |
| 13. Participation in recreation | | | | ✓ | ✓ |
| 14. Learning to satisfy curiosity | ✓ | | | ✓ | ✓ |

## SELECTING NURSING ACTIONS TO ASSIST A PATIENT WITH MULTIPLE DIFFICULTIES

We would now like you to choose from the list of Nursing Actions shown in *Table 7.2* those appropriate for Mrs Robinson during her recovery and rehabilitation period. Tick the appropriate columns and for each decision give an explanation for your choice. Then compare your choices of Nursing Action with those given on pages 210–211. Spaces will be left at the end of each living activity for other actions which you may feel are required.

*Table 7.2   Nursing actions to assist a patient who has difficulty with a number of living activities*

| Nursing actions | Yes | No | Maybe | Reason for choice |
|---|---|---|---|---|
| **Part 1 Breathing** | | | | |
| 1. Sit the patient upright | | | | |
| 2. Check patient's posture:<br>  (a) when sitting in bed<br>  (b) when sitting in chair | | | | |
| 3. Teach breathing exercises | | | | |
| 4. Give postural drainage | | | | |
| 5. Assist expectoration | | | | |
| 6. Provide:<br>  (a) sputum container<br>  (b) tissues<br>  (c) disposal bag | | | | |
| 7. Give oxygen | | | | |
| 8. Give steam inhalation | | | | |
| 9. Tell patient not to waste energy on doing breathing exercises | | | | |
| 10. ............................................. | | | | |
| 11. ............................................. | | | | |
| 12. ............................................. | | | | |
| **Part 2 Eating and Drinking** | | | | |
| 1. Provide normal diet | | | | |
| 2. Provide soft diet | | | | |
| 3. Provide liquid diet | | | | |
| 4. Assist in intravenous feeding | | | | |
| 5. Provide nasogastric feeding | | | | |

*Table 7.2    Continued*

| Nursing actions | Yes | No | Maybe | Reason for choice |
|---|---|---|---|---|
| **Part 2    Eating and Drinking (continued)** | | | | |
| 6. Give three large meals a day | | | | |
| 7. Give small frequent meals | | | | |
| 8. Help the patient to eat whatever she is able to manage | | | | |
| 9. Supplement meals on advice from dietician | | | | |
| 10. Provide reducing diet | | | | |
| 11. Give high fibre diet | | | | |
| 12. Give low residue diet | | | | |
| 13. Increase fluid intake | | | | |
| 14. Reduce fluid intake | | | | |
| 15. Encourage to sit at table with others at mealtimes | | | | |
| 16. Provide absolute privacy during mealtimes | | | | |
| 17. Cut up food for patient | | | | |
| 18. Seek guidance from occupational therapist for choice of appropriate eating aids | | | | |
| 19. Provide:<br>(a) non-slip table mat<br>(b) 'spoon and pusher'<br>(c) sharp knife | | | | |
| 20. Provide a bib | | | | |
| 21. Encourage staff in providing a sensitive and patient approach | | | | |
| 22. Encourage patient to complete meals in allotted time | | | | |
| 23. Ensure patient completes all that is offered | | | | |
| 24. Feed patient to save time | | | | |
| 25. Encourage relatives to bring favourite foods | | | | |
| 26. Check patient's posture throughout the meal | | | | |
| 27. Ensure utensils are within reach | | | | |

*Table 7.2  Continued*

| Nursing actions | Yes | No | Maybe | Reason for choice |
|---|---|---|---|---|
| **Part 2   Eating and Drinking (continued)** | | | | |
| 28. Attend to patient's mishaps promptly and kindly, e.g. spillages | | | | |
| 29. Ensure food is kept hot | | | | |
| 30.  Offer drinks with food | | | | |
| 31. Give assistance in choice of diet and menu orders | | | | |
| 32. Seek guidance from dietician in selecting appropriate diet | | | | |
| 33. ................................................. | | | | |
| 34. ................................................. | | | | |
| **Part 3 Eliminating** | | | | |
| 1. Give suppositories | | | | |
| 2. Give an enema/rectal washout | | | | |
| 3. Give an aperient | | | | |
| 4. Offer bedpans as required | | | | |
| 5. Offer commode as required | | | | |
| 6. Assist patient to lavatory:<br>(a) in wheelchair<br>(b) walking | | | | |
| 7. Stay with the patient while she is:<br>(a) using bedpan<br>(b) visiting the lavatory | | | | |
| 8. Assist with hygiene needs after elimination | | | | |
| 9. Provide raised lavatory seat | | | | |
| 10. Provide handrails in lavatory | | | | |
| 11. Ensure patient's privacy and warmth is maintained | | | | |
| 12. Attend to patient's mishaps promptly and kindly | | | | |
| 13. Provide incontinence pads | | | | |

*Table 7.2   Continued*

| Nursing actions | Yes | No | Maybe | Reason for choice |
|---|---|---|---|---|
| **Part 3   Eliminating (continued)** | | | | |
| 14. ................................................ | | | | |
| 15. ................................................ | | | | |
| 16. ................................................ | | | | |
| **Part 4 Sleeping and Resting** | | | | |
| 1. Offer a warm drink on settling at night | | | | |
| 2. Give prescribed night sedation | | | | |
| 3. Position patient's bed in a quiet area of the ward | | | | |
| 4. Position patient's bed near the lavatory | | | | |
| 5. Avoid making a noise near patient's bedside | | | | |
| 6. Minimise use of lights at night | | | | |
| 7. Make sure the ward is bright enough for patient to see the nurses | | | | |
| 8. Use a torch on patient's face to check patient is asleep | | | | |
| 9. Provide a call bell | | | | |
| 10. Place a commode at bedside | | | | |
| 11. Place a bedpan on a chair at the bedside | | | | |
| 12. Ensure ward area is well ventilated | | | | |
| 13. ................................................ | | | | |
| 14. ................................................ | | | | |
| **Part 5 Moving** | | | | |
| 1. Under direction of the physiotherapist, approach patient on affected side and assist patient to:<br>(a) move and sit in bed<br>(b) get out of bed into a chair<br>(c) move and sit in chair<br>(d) stand<br>(e) walk with aids if required<br>(f) climb stairs<br>(g) correct balance<br>   in bed<br>   in chair<br>   standing and walking<br>(h) use affected limbs in activities | | | | |

*Table 7.2    Continued*

| Nursing actions | Yes | No | Maybe | Reason for choice |
|---|---|---|---|---|
| **Part 5    Moving (continued)** | | | | |
| 2. Provide a mechanical hoist | | | | |
| 3. Turn patient from side to side while in bed | | | | |
| 4. Reposition affected limbs to prevent contractures and deformities | | | | |
| 5. Give passive exercises to affected limbs | | | | |
| 6. Lift patient in and out of bed | | | | |
| 7. Provide a sheepskin | | | | |
| 8. Keep patient at complete rest | | | | |
| 9. Under the direction of the occupational therapist, approach patient on affected side and assist patient to:<br>(a) dress and undress<br>(b) eat and drink<br>(c) prepare simple meals<br>(d) wash and bath<br>(e) care for hair using aids and encouraging use of affected limbs | | | | |
| 10. Provide hospital clothes | | | | |
| 11. Dress patient without her involvement | | | | |
| 12. Bath patient to save time | | | | |
| 13. Leave patient to bath herself | | | | |
| 14. Provide washing bowl at bedside | | | | |
| 15. Wash and set patient's hair | | | | |
| 16. Encourage constant activity throughout the day | | | | |
| 17. Provide opportunity for patient to rest during the day | | | | |
| 18. ................................................................. | | | | |
| 19. ................................................................. | | | | |
| **Part 6 Maintaining Body Temperature**<br>1. Provide light bedclothes | | | | |
| 2. Provide plenty of blankets | | | | |

*Table 7.2   Continued*

| Nursing actions | Yes | No | Maybe | Reason for choice |
|---|---|---|---|---|
| **Part 6   Maintaining Body Temperature (continued)**<br>3. Avoid chilling when sitting in a chair or visiting lavatory<br><br>4. Avoid exposure when in bed<br><br>5. ................................................ | | | | |
| **Part 7 Keeping Body Clean**<br>1. Give daily bed bath<br><br>2. Give daily bath in bathroom<br><br>3. Give weekly bath<br><br>4. Encourage patient to participate in:<br>  (a) washing<br>  (b) bathing<br>  (c) caring for hair<br>  (d) caring for nails<br>  (e) cleaning teeth<br><br>5. Provide opportunity for washing after elimination<br><br>6. Provide oral toilet 4-hourly<br><br>7. Cut patient's nails<br><br>8. Brush patient's hair<br><br>9. Encourage patient to continue using own personal deodorants, talcs, perfumes, soaps, bath foams/gels<br><br>10. ................................................<br><br>11. ................................................<br><br>12. ................................................ | | | | |
| **Part 8 Dressing Suitably**<br>1. Provide hospital nightdress<br><br>2. Provide hospital dressing gown and slippers<br><br>3. Encourage use of own night clothes<br><br>4. Encourage to be up and dressed in own clothes during the day | | | | |

*Table 7.2 Continued*

| Nursing actions | Yes | No | Maybe | Reason for choice |
|---|---|---|---|---|
| **Part 8 Dressing Suitably (continued)** | | | | |
| 5. Provide aids to prevent soiling of clothes | | | | |
| 6. Give guidance with the occupational therapist on alternative fastenings for dresses, coats, shoes, underwear | | | | |
| 7. Check the appropriateness of clothing for the environmental temperature and patient's activity level | | | | |
| 8. Wrap blankets firmly around patient when sitting in a chair | | | | |
| 9. Check the patient has someone to launder clothes | | | | |
| 10. Help patient to change clothes if soiled | | | | |
| 11. Ignore patient's wishes regarding choice of clothes | | | | |
| 12. ................................ | | | | |
| 13. ................................ | | | | |
| 14. ................................ | | | | |
| **Part 9 Avoiding Danger and Injury** | | | | |
| 1. Position locker within reach of affected side | | | | |
| 2. Position locker out of reach | | | | |
| 3. Provide a call bell: (a) in bathroom (b) in lavatory (c) at bedside | | | | |
| 4. Fix cotsides: (a) during the day (b) during the night | | | | |
| 5. Anticipate patient's need for help | | | | |
| 6. Check ward floor is free from spillages | | | | |
| 7. Allow patient to walk unaided | | | | |
| 8. Discuss with relatives the need for suitable footwear | | | | |

*Table 7.2   Continued*

| Nursing actions | Yes | No | Maybe | Reason for choice |
|---|---|---|---|---|
| **Part 9 Avoiding Danger and Injury (continued)** | | | | |
| 9. Teach the patient how to avoid ward hazards, i.e. <br>(a) floor cleaning <br>(b) movement of staff and equipment | | | | |
| 10. Encourage patient's awareness of risks involved in use of affected limbs | | | | |
| 11. Ensure staff are aware of potential risks to this patient | | | | |
| 12. ................................................................ | | | | |
| 13. ................................................................ | | | | |
| 14. ................................................................ | | | | |
| **Part 10 Communicating** | | | | |
| 1. Provide a call bell: <br>(a) at bedside <br>(b) in bathroom <br>(c) in lavatory <br>(d) in day room | | | | |
| 2. Provide picture/word cards | | | | |
| 3. Provide notepad and pencil | | | | |
| 4. Allocate a nurse to establish a relationship | | | | |
| 5. Allocate time to assist patient to speak, under the guidance of the speech therapist | | | | |
| 6. Ensure that the nursing team do not misinterpret patient's non-verbal cues | | | | |
| 7. Complete patient's words/sentences for her | | | | |
| 8. Raise voice when talking to patient | | | | |
| 9. Choose questions to elicit responses within the patient's ability | | | | |
| 10. Give directions to patient which need no response | | | | |
| 11. Avoid discussing prognosis with patient | | | | |
| 12. Keep patient informed of progress, changes and plans | | | | |

*Table 7.2  Continued*

| Nursing actions | Yes | No | Maybe | Reason for choice |
|---|---|---|---|---|
| **Part 10  Communicating (continued)** | | | | |
| 13. Gain patient's views and allow participation in decision-making | | | | |
| 14. ................................................. | | | | |
| 15. ................................................. | | | | |
| 16. ................................................. | | | | |
| **Part 11 Worshipping** | | | | |
| 1. Inform hospital chaplain of patient's admission | | | | |
| 2. Inform patient's own chaplain | | | | |
| 3. Ignore patient's requests to attend Chapel | | | | |
| 4. Contact chaplain if patient requests Holy Communion on the ward | | | | |
| 5. Provide opportunities for communal worship within the ward | | | | |
| 6. Encourage use of hospital religious broadcasts | | | | |
| 7. ................................................. | | | | |
| 8. ................................................. | | | | |
| **Part 12 Working** | | | | |
| 1. Arrange for home assessment by the occupational therapist | | | | |
| 2. Assume relatives will take over shopping/ cooking/housework | | | | |
| 3. Allow discharge prior to modification of home without assistance from others | | | | |
| 4. Arrange for home care assistant for shopping and housework | | | | |
| 5. ................................................. | | | | |
| 6. ................................................. | | | | |
| **Part 13 Participating in Recreation** | | | | |
| 1. Assist in choosing suitable diversional therapy | | | | |

*Table 7.2 Continued*

| Nursing actions | Yes | No | Maybe | Reason for choice |
|---|---|---|---|---|
| **Part 13 Participating in Recreation (continued)**<br><br>2. Show an interest in patient's own activities<br><br>3. Encourage the patient in physical exercise to improve coordination<br><br>4. Read patient's personal mail to her<br><br>5. Assist patient in using the television room/ reading daily papers<br><br>6. All recreational activities to cease after 11 pm to ensure a good night's sleep<br><br>7. ................................................<br><br>8. ................................................ | | | | |
| **Part 14 Learning and Satisfying Curiosity**<br>1. Keep the patient and relations fully informed of her progress and condition<br><br>2. Avoid discussing long-term expectations<br><br>3. Make sure that ward staff are kept fully informed about explanations given to the patient and relatives<br><br>4. Provide opportunity for patient and relatives to meet medical and paramedical staff<br><br>5. ................................................<br><br>6. ................................................ | | | | |

## CHOICE OF NURSING ACTIONS

We have made the following choices. If yours differ from ours, check you reasons for choice and be prepared to discuss your reasoning with colleague and staff. You may have found from your own experience that other Nursin Actions may be appropriate and spaces have been provided for you to mak additions.

Part 1   Yes   Numbers 2(a) and (b), 3
          No     Numbers 7, 8 and 9
          Maybe Numbers 1, 4, 5, 6(a), (b) and (c)
Part 2   Yes   Numbers 7, 8, 9, 11, 15, 18, 21, 26, 27, 28, 29, 31, 32
          No     Numbers 4, 5, 6, 12, 14, 19(c), 20, 23, 24
          Maybe Numbers 1, 2, 3, 10, 13, 16, 17, 19(a) and (b), 22, 25, 30

Part 3  Yes    Numbers 4, 5, 6(a), 8, 9, 10, 11, 12
        No     Number  2
        Maybe  Numbers 1, 3, 6(b) and (c), 7(a) and (b), 13
Part 4  Yes    Numbers 1, 3, 4, 5, 6, 9, 12
        No     Numbers 8, 11
        Maybe  Numbers 2, 7, 10
Part 5  Yes    Numbers 1(a), (b), (c), (d), (e), (g), (h), 4, 9(a), (b), (d), (e), 17
        No     Numbers 8, 11, 12, 13, 14, 16
        Maybe  Numbers 1(f), 2, 3, 5, 6, 7, 9(c), 10, 15
Part 6  Yes    Numbers 3, 4
        No     —
        Maybe  Numbers 1, 2
Part 7  Yes    Numbers 4(a), (b), (c), (d), (e), 5, 9
        No     Number  6
        Maybe  Numbers 1, 2, 3, 7, 8
Part 8  Yes    Numbers 3, 4, 6, 7, 9, 10
        No     Numbers 8, 11
        Maybe  Numbers 1, 2, 5
Part 9  Yes    Numbers 1, 3(a), (b), (c), 5, 6, 8, 9, 10, 11
        No     Number  2
        Maybe  Numbers 4(a), (b), 7
Part 10 Yes    Numbers 1(a), (b), (c), (d), 4, 5, 6, 9, 12, 13
        No     Numbers 7, 8, 10, 11
        Maybe  Numbers 2, 3
Part 11 Yes    Numbers 4, 5, 6
        No     Number  3
        Maybe  Numbers 1, 2
Part 12 Yes    Number  1
        No     Numbers 2, 3
        Maybe  Number  4
Part 13 Yes    Numbers 1, 2, 3, 5
        No     Number  6
        Maybe  Number  4
Part 14 Yes    Numbers 1, 3, 4
        No     Number  2
        Maybe  —

We now ask you to identify priorities for planning the care that Mrs Robinson requires to help her with her difficulties in a number of living activities.

## CHOOSING PRIORITIES IN NURSING ACTIONS

*Table 7.3   Priorities in nursing actions*

| Part | Insert your choice of priority numbers 1–14 |
|------|---------------------------------------------|
| 1. Breathing | |
| 2. Eating and drinking | |
| 3. Eliminating | |
| 4. Sleeping and resting | |
| 5. Moving | |
| 6. Maintaining body temperature | |
| 7. Keeping body clean | |
| 8. Dressing suitably | |
| 9. Avoiding danger and injury | |
| 10. Communicating | |
| 11. Worshipping | |
| 12. Working | |
| 13. Participating in recreation | |
| 14. Learning to satisfy curiosity | |

You can check your decision regarding priority choice of nursing actions with the plan shown in *Table 7.4*. If you wish to remind yourself about planning and providing nursing care please refer again to *Figure 3.4*, Chapter 3.

## IDENTIFICATION OF CRITERIA FOR PROGRESS

You should now read carefully the plan shown in *Table 7.4* which identifies criteria for progress.

*Table 7.4 Plan of care for progress*

| Nursing actions to assist a patient with a number of living activities | Yes | Maybe | Priority Choice | Measurements | Short-term goals | Review period | Evaluation Criteria Have short-term goals been met? |
|---|---|---|---|---|---|---|---|
| **Part 9 Avoiding Dangers and Injury** | | | | Record and report: Potential hazards in ward area | No incident or accident occurs to the patient | On-going | No incidents or accidents but patient requires close supervision |
| 1. Position locker within reach | ✓ | | | spillages obstacles congestion | | | |
| 3. Provide a call bell: (a) in bathroom | ✓ | | | Check patient's awareness of | | | |
| (b) in lavatory | ✓ | | | limitations and abilities in | | | |
| (c) at bedside | ✓ | | | moving coping with living | | | |
| 4. Fix cotsides: (a) during the day | | ✓ | | activities | | | |
| (b) during the night | | ✓ | | | | | |
| 5. Anticipate patient's need for help | ✓ | | | | | | |
| 6. Check ward floor is free from spillages | ✓ | | | | | | |
| 7. Allow patient to walk unaided | | ✓ | FIRST | | | | |
| 8. Discuss with relatives the need for suitable footwear | ✓ | | | | | | |
| 9. Teach the patient how to avoid ward hazards, i.e. (a) floor cleaning | ✓ | | | | | | |
| (b) movement of staff and equipment | ✓ | | | | | | |
| 10. Encourage patient's awareness of risks involved in the use of affected limbs | ✓ | | | | | | |
| 11. Ensure staff are aware of potential risks to this patient | ✓ | | | | | | |
| **Part 6 Maintaining Body Temperature** | | | | Note when patient complains of feeling hot or cold | Patient feels comfortable | On-going | Requires extra protection when using bathroom |
| 1. Provide light bedclothes | | ✓ | | Measure and record body temperature 12-hourly | Body temperature remains within normal limits | 24-hourly | Within normal limits |
| 2. Provide plenty of blankets | | ✓ | SECOND | | | | |
| 3. Avoid chilling when sitting in a chair or visiting lavatory | ✓ | | | | | | |

*Table 7.4   Continued*

| Nursing actions to assist a patient with a number of living difficulties. | Yes | Maybe | Priority Choice | Measurements | Short-term goals | Review period | Evaluation Criteria Have short-term goals been met? |
|---|---|---|---|---|---|---|---|
| **Part 6   Maintaining Body Temperature (continued)** | | | S E C O N D | | | | |
| 4. Avoid exposure when in bed | ✓ | | | | | | |
| **Part 2   Eating and Drinking** | | | | Record: | (a), (b), (c), (d) Intake of 2 litres of fluid | 8-hourly | Has drunk 1 litre only and consumed 1500 calories, soft diet. Does not take sugar in beverages |
| 1. Provide normal diet | | ✓ | | (a) How much food and fluid is eaten and drunk | | | |
| 2. Provide soft diet | | ✓ | | | and | | |
| 3. Provide liquid diet | | ✓ | | (b) Frequency of taking food and drink | 1,500 calories in 24 hours | | |
| 7. Give small frequent meals | ✓ | | | | | | |
| 8. Help the patient to eat whatever she is able to manage | ✓ | | | (c) When she feels hungry | Not feeling hungry | | Does not appear to be hungry |
| 9. Supplement meals on advice from dietician | ✓ | | | (d) Type of intake—likes and dislikes | | | |
| 10. Provide reducing diet | | ✓ | | (e) Weight | Maintain present weight | Weekly | Not weighed yet |
| 11. Give high fibre diet | ✓ | | | (f) Difficulty In chewing and swallowing | Able to return to normal diet | On-going | Manages soft foods only |
| 13. Increase fluid intake | | ✓ | | Note any distress when eating with others | Able to socialise at mealtimes | At meal-times | Anxious because she takes longer to eat |
| 15. Encourage to sit at table with others at mealtimes | ✓ | | T H I R D | | | | |
| 16. Provide absolute privacy during mealtimes | | ✓ | | | | | |
| 17. Cut up food for patient | | ✓ | | | | | |
| 18. Seek guidance from occupational therapist for choice of appropriate eating aids | ✓ | | | | | | |
| 19. Provide (a) non-slip table mat and | ✓ | | | | | | |
| (b) 'spoon and pusher' | ✓ | | | | | | |
| 21. Encourage staff in providing a sensitive and patient approach | ✓ | | | | | | |

*Table 7.4 Continued*

| Nursing actions to assist a patient with a number of living activities | Yes | Maybe | Priority Choice | Measurements | Short-term goals | Review period | Evaluation Criteria Have short-term goals been met? |
|---|---|---|---|---|---|---|---|
| **Part 2 Eating and Drinking (continued)** | | | THIRD | | | | |
| 22. Encourage patient to complete meals in allotted time | | ✓ | | | | | |
| 25. Encourage relatives to bring favourite foods | | ✓ | | | | | |
| 26. Check patient's posture throughout the meal | ✓ | | | | | | |
| 27. Ensure utensils are within reach | ✓ | | | | | | |
| 28. Attend to patient's mishaps promptly and kindly, e.g. spillages | ✓ | | | | | | |
| 29. Ensure food is kept hot | ✓ | | | | | | |
| 30. Offer drinks with food | | ✓ | | | | | |
| 31. Give assistance in choice of diet and menu orders | ✓ | | | | | | |
| 32. Seek guidance from dietician to selecting appropriate diet | ✓ | | | | | | |
| **Part 5 Moving** | | | FOURTH | Note signs and symptoms of complications of immobility: | | | |
| 1. Under direction of the physiotherapist, assist patient to: | | | | | | | |
| (a) move and sit in bed | ✓ | | | (a) Temperature, pulse, respiration and local signs of infection, e.g. chest infection or urinary tract infection | (a) Prevent infection or detect early | 4-hourly | Within normal limits |
| (b) get out of bed into a chair | ✓ | | | | | | |
| (c) move and sit in chair | ✓ | | | | | | |
| (d) stand | ✓ | | | (b) Presence of redness or abrasions on pressure sites | (b) Pressure areas remain intact | 4-hourly | Intact |
| (e) walk, with aids if required | ✓ | | | | | | |
| (f) climb stairs | | ✓ | | | | | |
| (g) correct balance in bed | ✓ | | | (c) Range of movement of limbs and joints | (c) Full range maintained | 24-hourly | Full range possible on affected side |
| in chair | ✓ | | | | | | |
| standing and walking | ✓ | | | (d) Sensation in limbs | (d) No injuries while sensations impaired | 24-hourly | Tingling in leg, arm anaesthetic |
| (h) use affected limbs in activities | ✓ | | | | | | |

*Table 7.4   Continued*

| Nursing actions to assist a patient with a number of living activities | Yes | Maybe | Priority Choice | Measurements | Short-term goals | Review period | Evaluation Criteria Have short-term goals been met? |
|---|---|---|---|---|---|---|---|
| **Part 5   Moving (continued)** | | | ⎤ | (e) Signs of muscle wasting, contractures, drop foot, stiffness | (e) Prevent or detect early signs | 24-hourly | No obvious muscle wasting. Some stiffness in knee |
| 2. Provide a mechanical hoist | | ✓ | | | | | |
| 3. Turn patient from side to side while in bed | | ✓ | | (f) Muscle tone and power | (f) Protect affected limbs | On-going | Arm—flaccid paralysis Leg—some spasticity |
| 4. Reposition affected limbs to prevent contractures and deformities | ✓ | | | Report changes in use of aids, e.g. walking frame, sticks | Enable increasing independence | On-going | Able to stand with walking frame. Starting to hold spoon and feed herself with unaffected hand |
| 5. Give passive exercises to affected limbs | | ✓ | | | | | |
| 6. Lift patient in and out of bed | | ✓ | | | | | |
| 7. Provide a sheepskin | | ✓ | FOURTH | | | | |
| 9. Under the direction of the occupational therapist, assist patient to: | ✓ | | | | | | |
| (a) dress and undress | ✓ | | | | | | |
| (b) eat and drink | ✓ | | | | | | |
| (c) prepare simple meals | | ✓ | | | | | |
| (d) wash and bath | ✓ | | | | | | |
| (e) care for hair using aids | ✓ | | | | | | |
| (f) encourage use of affected limbs in personal care | ✓ | | | | | | |
| 10. Provide hospital clothes | | ✓ | | | | | |
| 15. Wash and set patient's hair; visit hairdresser | | ✓ | | | | | |
| 17. Provide opportunity for patient to rest during the day | ✓ | | ⎦ | | | | |
| **Part 1   Breathing** | | | ⎤ | Measure and record: Rate and depth of respiration | Normal effortless breathing | 4-hourly | Respirations normal Tends to slump to one side impeding full chest expansion |
| 1. Sit the patient upright | | ✓ | FIFTH | | | | |
| 2. Check patient's posture | | | | Note: Colour Difficulty with breathing sputum | No sputum | | No cough or sputum |
| (a) when sitting in bed | ✓ | | | | | | |
| (b) when sitting in chair | ✓ | | ⎦ | | | | |

*Table 7.4  Continued*

| Nursing actions to assist a patient with a number of living activities | Yes | Maybe | Priority Choice | Measurements | Short-term goals | Review period | Evaluation Criteria Have short-term goals been met? |
|---|---|---|---|---|---|---|---|
| **Part 1  Breathing (continued)** | | | | | | | |
| 3. Teach breathing exercises | ✓ | | FIFTH | | | | |
| 4. Give postural drainage | | ✓ | | | | | |
| 5. Assist expectoration | | ✓ | | | | | |
| 6. Provide (a) sputum container | | ✓ | | | | | |
| (b) tissues | | ✓ | | | | | |
| (c) disposal bag | | ✓ | | | | | |
| **Part 10 Communicating** | | | SIXTH | Note level of anxiety and/or frustration from patient and relatives | Patient and relatives are confident in care being given | On-going | Mrs Robinson seems fully aware of the implications of treatment and length of stay in hospital |
| 1. Provide a call bell at bedside | ✓ | | | | | | |
| in bathroom | ✓ | | | Note ability to form words, sentences | Able to speak using simple sentences | Twice weekly | |
| in lavatory | ✓ | | | | | | |
| in day room | ✓ | | | Note appropriateness of response to questions | Attempting to respond | | |
| 2. Provide picture/ word cards | | ✓ | | | | | |
| 3. Provide notepad and pencil | | ✓ | | Note whether patient and/or relatives become uncommunicative, withdrawn, depressed, over-anxious | | On-going | Exhibiting the expected response to her condition, i.e. concerned but not over-anxious |
| 4. Allocate a nurse to establish a relationship | ✓ | | | | | | |
| 5. Allocate time to assist patient to speak, under the guidance of the speech therapist | ✓ | | | | | | |
| 6. Ensure the nursing team do not misinterpret patient's non-verbal cues | ✓ | | | | | | |
| 9. Choose questions to elicit responses within the patient's ability | ✓ | | | | | | |
| 12. Keep patient informed of progress, changes and plans | ✓ | | | | | | |
| 13. Gain patient's views and allow participation in decision-making | ✓ | | | | | | |

*Table 7.4   Continued*

| Nursing actions to assist a patient with a number of living activities | Yes | Maybe | Priority Choice | Measurements | Short-term goals | Review period | Evaluation Criteria Have short-term goals been met? |
|---|---|---|---|---|---|---|---|
| **Part 14   Learning and Satisfying Curiosity** | | | *(SIXTH)* | Note: Mrs Robinson's orientation to time and place | Orientated to present setting | On-going | Fully orientated to ward setting but not yet interested in events outside |
| 1. Keep the patient and relations fully informed of her progress and condition | ✓ | | | Any queries from patient or relatives | Queries dealt with as they occur | On-going | |
| 3. Make sure that ward staff are kept fully informed about explanations given to the patient and relatives | ✓ | | | | | | |
| 4. Provide opportunity for patient and relatives to meet medical and paramedical staff | ✓ | | | | | | |
| **Part 3   Eliminating** | | | *(SEVENTH)* | (a) Measure and record fluid output | (a) Output of 1500 ml of urine in 24 hours | 12-hourly | (a) Output 1000 ml only |
| 1. Give suppositories | | ✓ | | | | | |
| 3. Give an aperient | | ✓ | | (b) Note frequency, pain, urgency of micturition | (b) Infection free, normal filling and emptying of bladder | On-going | (b) Some urgency of micturition |
| 4. Offer bedpan when required | ✓ | | | | | | |
| 5. Offer commode when required | ✓ | | | (c) Test urine for presence of albumin, blood, glucose, bile | (c) Normal urine | If abnormalities occur | (c) No abnormalities detected |
| 6. Assist patient to lavatory: | ✓ | | | | | | |
| (a) in wheelchair | | ✓ | | (d) Note level of independence achieved | (d) Continent, minimal assistance | On-going | (d) Continent, needs assistance to get to the lavatory |
| (b) to walk | | ✓ | | | | | |
| 7. Stay with the patient while she is: | | | | | | | Requires bedpan occasionally and at night. Needs help with re-adjusting clothing |
| (a) using bedpan | | ✓ | | | | | |
| (b) visiting the lavatory | | ✓ | | | | | |
| 8. Assist with hygiene needs following elimination | ✓ | | | (e) Note consistency and frequency of bowel action | (e) Restoration of normal bowel function | 24-hourly | (e) No bowel action for past 48 hours |
| 9. Provide raised lavatory seat | ✓ | | | | | | |
| 10. Provide handrails in lavatory | ✓ | | | | | | |
| 11. Ensure patient's privacy and warmth is maintained | ✓ | | | | | | |
| 12. Attend to patient's mishaps promptly and kindly | ✓ | | | | | | |

*Table 7.4    Continued*

| Nursing actions to assist a patient with a number of living activities | Yes | Maybe | Priority Choice | Measurements | Short-term goals | Review period | Evaluation Criteria Have short-term goals been met? |
|---|---|---|---|---|---|---|---|
| **Part 3   Eliminating (continued)** 13. Provide incontinence pads | | ✓ | }SEVENTH | | | | |
| **Part 4   Sleeping and Resting** 1. Offer a warm drink on settling at night | ✓ | | | Record: (a) Length of sleep (b) Number of disturbances during the night (c) If disturbed, what has woken her (d) Whether she wakes refreshed (e) Whether night sedation is required | 6-7 hours total sleep or rest during the night | 24-hourly | Disturbed by requiring change of position Wakes early, not fully refreshed. Requires rest periods during the day Night sedation refused |
| 2. Give prescribed night sedation | | ✓ | | | | | |
| 3. Position patient's bed in a quiet area of the ward | ✓ | | | | | | |
| 4. Position patient's bed near the lavatory | ✓ | | | | | | |
| 5. Avoid making a noise near patient's bedside | ✓ | | | | | | |
| 6. Minimise use of lights at night | ✓ | | | | | | |
| 7. Make sure the ward is light enough for patient to see the nurses | | ✓ | }EIGHTH | | | | |
| 9. Provide a call bell | ✓ | | | | | | |
| 10. Place a commode at bedside | | ✓ | | | | | |
| 12. Ensure ward area is well ventilated | ✓ | | | | | | |
| **Part 11   Worshipping** 1. Inform hospital chaplain of patient's admission | | ✓ | | Note Mrs Robinson's desire for spiritual help | Satisfaction of spiritual needs if necessary | On-going | Would like to attend hospital chapel services |
| 2. Inform patient's own chaplain | | ✓ | | | | | |
| 4. Contact chaplain if patient requests Holy Communion on the ward | ✓ | | | | | | |
| 5. Provide opportunities for communal worship within the ward | ✓ | | | | | | |

*Table 7.4 Continued*

| Nursing actions to assist a patient with a number of living activities | Yes | Maybe | Priority Choice | Measurements | Short-term goals | Review period | Evaluation Criteria Have short-term goals been met? |
|---|---|---|---|---|---|---|---|
| **Part 11 Worshipping (continued)** | | | ⌐ EIGHTH ⌐ | | | | |
| 6. Encourage use of hospital religious broadcasts | ✓ | | | | | | |
| **Part 13 Participating in Recreation** | | | | Note how Mrs Robinson is occupied during the day | Provide suitable stimulus if required | 24-hourly | Social and physical rehabilitation programme takes all her energies at present |
| 1. Assist in choosing suitable diversional therapy | ✓ | | | | | | |
| 2. Show an interest in patient's own activities | ✓ | | | | | | |
| 3. Encourage the patient in physical exercise to improve coordination | ✓ | | | | | | |
| 4. Read patient's personal mail to her | | ✓ | | | | | |
| 5. Assist patient in using the television room/reading daily papers | ✓ | | | | | | |
| **Part 7 Keeping Body Clean** | | | ⌐ NINTH ⌐ | (a) Note patient's ability to cope with her own hygiene | (a) Maintain cleanliness during period of partial dependence | 24-hourly | (a) Still requires considerable assistance with washing and bathing. Mechanical hoist needed for bathing |
| 1. Give daily bed bath | | ✓ | | | | | |
| 2. Give daily bath in bathroom | | ✓ | | | | | |
| 3. Give weekly bath | | ✓ | | | | | |
| 4. Encourage patient to participate in: (a) washing (b) bathing (c) caring for hair (d) caring for nails (e) cleaning teeth | ✓ ✓ ✓ ✓ ✓ | | | (b) Note state of skin, mouth, hair, and nails | (b) Maintain care of skin, mouth, teeth, hair and nails | 8-hourly | (b) Skin intact, well cared for. Mouth moist, no cracks or abrasions. Hair requires shampooing |
| 5. Provide opportunity for washing after elimination | ✓ | | | | | | |
| 7. Cut patient's nails | | ✓ | | | | | |
| 8. Brush patient's hair | | ✓ | | | | | |

*Table 7.4  Continued*

| Nursing actions to assist a patient with a number of living activities | Yes | Maybe | Priority Choice | Measurements | Short-term goals | Review period | Evaluation Criteria Have short-term goals been met? |
|---|---|---|---|---|---|---|---|
| **Part 7   Keeping Body Clean (continued)** | | | | | | | |
| 9. Encourage patient to continue using own personal deodorants, talcs, perfumes, soaps, bath foams/gels | ✓ | | | | | | |
| **Part 8   Dressing Suitably** | | | | (a) Note patient's ability to undress and dress, manage buttons and fastenings | (a) Patient able to participate in dressing and undressing | On-going | (a) Is taking an active interest in attempting to dress, selects clothes but is unable to dress |
| 1. Provide hospital nightdress | | ✓ | | | | | |
| 2. Provide hospital dressing gown and slippers | | ✓ | | (b) Note that patient is dressed appropriately to her body temperature, environment and level of activity | (b) Patient not overheated or chilled | 4-hourly | (b) Tends to get cold when moving from one area to another |
| 3. Encourage use of own night clothes | ✓ | | | | | | |
| 4. Encourage to be up and dressed in own clothes during the day | ✓ | | | | | | |
| 5. Provide aids to prevent soiling of clothes | | ✓ | | | | | |
| 6. Give guidance with the occupational therapist on alternative fastenings for dresses, coats, shoes, underwear | ✓ | | | | | | |
| 7. Check the appropriateness of clothing for the temperature and patient's activity level | ✓ | | | | | | |
| 9. Check that patient has someone to launder clothes | ✓ | | | | | | |
| 10. Help patient to change clothes if soiled | ✓ | | | | | | |

(Priority Choice column, spanning bracket: NINTH)

*Table 7.4  Continued*

| Nursing actions to assist a patient with a number of living activities | Yes | Maybe | Priority Choice | Measurements | Short-term goals | Review period | Evaluation Criteria Have short-term goals been met? |
|---|---|---|---|---|---|---|---|
| **Part 12  Working**<br>1. Arrange for home assessment by the occupational therapist<br><br>4. Arrange for home care assistant for shopping and housework | ✓ | ✓ | TENTH | Home assessment: check ability of family to support Mrs Robinson | Prepare for discharge home | On-going | Early discussions with occupational therapist, social worker, district nurse, relatives, GP, voluntary services |

### *Using Evaluation Criteria for Resetting Short-term Goals*

We have again given you an example of care planning and use of evaluation criteria for resetting short-term goals. This may mean consideration of changing measurements and review periods as Mrs Robinson's progress alters and new short-term goals are identified.

### IDENTIFICATION OF LONG-TERM GOALS

As a final exercise we would like you to set long-term goals for Mrs Robinson assuming that she will be independent enough to return home but with some assistance due to residual weakness on her affected side.

To assist you in preparing a long-term goal profile we suggest you use the following example profiles to help you to decide how her physiological, security, achievement and self-fulfilment needs might be met: Section 1, profiles 9, 12, 14, 15, 18, together with the plan shown in *Figure 7.13*.

**Figure 7.13** *Long-term goal profile for Mrs Robinson*

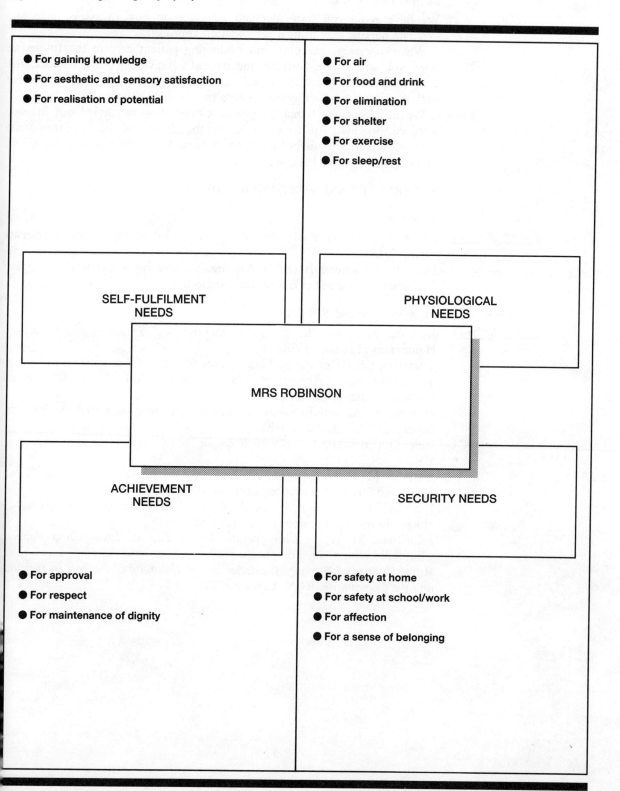

## SUMMARY NOTES

We have given you some detailed guidance on how to assess, plan and evaluate nursing care using a personalised approach.

When assessing, planning and evaluating patient care in the future we hope you will always consider the patient's individual characteristics, i.e. age, temperament, social/cultural setting and capacity as well as his/her pathological state affecting basic needs that require assistance.

We do not suggest that lengthy documentation is carried out in each instance, provided you have considered the above and the resources available. However, you might like to check periodically the care you are giving by using the tools we have suggested.

## REFERENCES AND FURTHER READING

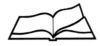

### References

Green, J. H. (1978). *Basic Clinical Physiology*, 3rd edition. Oxford University Press, Oxford.

Hunt, P. and Sendell, B. (1987). *Nursing the Adult with a Specific Physiological Disturbance*. Macmillan Education, London.

### Suggested Further Reading

Bobath, B. *Adult Hemiplegia Evaluation and Treatment*, 2nd edition. Heinemann, London, 1978.

Chartered Society of Physiotherapy. *Handling the Handicapped: A Guide to the Lifting and Movement of Disabled People*, 2nd edition. Woodhead-Faulkner, Cambridge, 1980.

Downie, P. A. and Kennedy, P. *Lifting, Handling and Helping Patients*. Faber and Faber, London, 1981.

Hale, G. (Ed.). *The New Source Book for the Disabled*. Heinemann, London, 1983.

Hawker, M. *Return to Mobility: Exercises for Stroke Patients*. The Chest, Heart and Stroke Association, London, 1978.

Isted, C. R. *Learning to Speak Again After a Stroke*. King Edward's Hospital Fund for London, London, 1979.

Johnstone, M. *Home Care for the Stroke Patient: Living in a Pattern*. Churchill Livingstone, Edinburgh, 1980.

Royal College of Nursing. *Guidance on the Handling of Patients in Hospital and the Community*. RCN, London, 1983.

# Section 3　The Nurse

## Introduction

In this final section we are going to look at some of the roles of the nurse in his/her attempts to give personalised care. We have chosen to look at the Nurse as a

- Giver of care
- Friend, counsellor/helper
- Facilitator
- Assessor
- Planner
- Teacher
- Manager
- Evaluator
- Researcher

We would like you to consider how you incorporate each of these functions into your daily work by attempting to answer the pertinent questions on each page. We hope you will find these useful as a means of self-assessment or as a basis for discussion with your colleagues or as suggestions for written work, seminars or debates. This is not to suggest that there are any definite right or wrong answers but rather that the value to be gained is in the thought given to the questions as your knowledge, skills and experience develop.

There may be other roles you may wish to add, consider and discuss with your colleagues. We are using this section to encourage you to think in some depth about the various roles of the nurse. For further thought you may like to use the list of suggested reading at the end of Chapter 8.

# Chapter 8
# The Roles of the Nurse

The roles of the nurse are described below in diagrammatic form, with questions to act as a framework for your discussion and evaluation.

**Figure 8.1**  *The nurse as a giver of care*

Do you like to plan your work?

Do you think nurses should become involved in their patients' problems?

THE NURSE
AS A GIVER OF CARE

Do you think your patients should be dependent on you?

Do you like to involve your patient:
● In planning care?
● In giving care?
● In evaluating care?

How skilled are you in giving care?
● Do you seek guidance/
  support if certain
  skills are new to you?
● How do you keep up to date?
● Do you seek appraisal of your skills
  from the patient?
  from your colleagues?

Do you think the nurse should be the only health worker/professional involved in meeting a patient's needs?

**Figure 8.2**   *The nurse as a friend, counsellor/helper*

Do you tell patients what to do?

Do you assist the patient in interacting with other professionals?

Do you listen to patients?

Do you get upset when a patient leaves your care?

Do you provide privacy?

**THE NURSE AS A FRIEND, COUNSELLOR/HELPER**

Do you listen to relatives?

Do you recognise when your patient is upset/anxious?

Do you return to your patients after interruptions?

Do you avoid the unpopular patient?

Do you know when to respect the patient's confidence and when to refer to others?

How are you going to maintain the helping relationship in the long term?

**Figure 8.3** *The nurse as a facilitator*

How do you facilitate
- communication
- liaison
- learning
- caring
- planning
- evaluating
- assessing?

How good are you at interacting with others?
- Do you greet people warmly?
- Can you assist others to participate?
- Do you listen to other people's views?

**THE NURSE AS A FACILITATOR**

How do you assess needs of:
- patients
- relatives
- students
- staff
- others?

Are you prepared to provide resources for others to carry out their ideas?

What resources have you available to meet needs?
- specialist knowledge, skills
- a learning environment

How approachable are you to others?
- Do people come to you with difficulties, suggestions and ideas?

**Figure 8.4** *The nurse as an assessor*

Do you take into consideration:
● The individual patient's physical and mental abilities?

How do you measure against standards?

Do you take into consideration:
● stage of training
● previous experience
● knowledge
● need for encouragement and praise
● need for future assistance?

What standards do you use?

THE NURSE AS AN ASSESSOR

Do you consider the physical environment?
● space
● heating
● lighting

What can alter your perception of events?
● Your past experiences
● Your attitudes
● Your observation skills
● Your analytical skills
● Your objectivity/subjectivity

What biases and prejudices do you possess?

Can your biases and prejudices affect how you assess others?

**Figure 8.5**   *The nurse as a planner*

Do you define the problem?

How do you consider options, choices?

How do you allocate your resources?

THE NURSE AS A PLANNER

Do you set yourself short- and long-term goals?

Do you ever make contingency plans?

Do you set yourself a time limit?

How do you analyse a problem?

Do you ever seek expert advice?

Do you involve others in planning?
● patient
● relatives
● colleagues
● others

**Figure 8.6** *The nurse as a teacher*

Who do you think requires teaching from you in your ward/unit?

How do you know you have been a successful teacher?

How do you engender a climate for learning?

How would you teach a member of the domestic staff the reasons for barrier nursing precaution for a patient in your ward?

How do you teach?
● by example
● by telling
● by discussing
● by showing
● by offering supervision
● by giving opportunities

## THE NURSE AS A TEACHER

Do you think teaching should only take place in a classroom?

When would you consider teaching a relative how to care for a patient's hygiene?
● in afternoon's rest period
● the day of discharge
● when normally hygiene needs are attended to

How could one of your patients learn to give an injection?
● by trial and error
● by being told
● by being shown
● by long practice

How do you know if a patient, relative, student or other staff are ill informed?

**Figure 8.7** *The nurse as a manager*

How do you lead?
- by setting clear objectives
- by example
- by involvement with staff
- by enforcing discipline
- by generating enthusiasm

How do you initiate change?
- by imposition
- by encouraging involvement
- by asking someone else to do it

How do you set priorities?

## THE NURSE AS A MANAGER

What sort of Manager are you?
- Do you delegate your work?
- Do you discuss problems with your staff?
- Do you encourage your staff to make suggestions?
- Do you tell your staff what you expect from them?

How do you liaise with others?
- formally
- informally
- regularly
- as the need arises
- when asked by others

Do you obtain the patient/client viewpoint?

How much do you plan ahead?
- for duty rostas for holidays
- for ward organisation
- for ordering supplies
- for changes in staff

How do you monitor?
- quality of patient care
- staff relationships
- use of equipment
- other resources

**Figure 8.8** *The nurse as an evaluator*

How are you going to decide on which measurement tools to use?

How do you cope with negative results?
● Do you reject/alter/ignore?
● Do reappraisal?
● Do you involve others?
● Do you change your plans?

How are you going to provide feedback of results?

**THE NURSE AS AN EVALUATOR**

What parameters do you set?

What do you use as a baseline for deciding standards?

What do you do with the results?
● Do you allow discussion?
● With whom do you discuss?
● Do you reset goals?

**Figure 8.9** *The nurse as a researcher*

Are you aware of current research in your field of work?
If not, why not? Is it due to
● lack of resources
● lack of opportunity
● lack of interest?

What would you do with your research findings on completion of a research project?

Do you think nursing is research based?

## THE NURSE AS A RESEARCHER

If you could carry out a piece of research what would this be?

Is the patient/nurse/relationship altered during observation studies?

What skills are developed when carrying out a piece of research?

Are you currently introducing nursing research findings into your patient care?

Should nurses be researchers?

What is preventing you carrying out a research project on your ward?

Should the patient be asked if he/she wishes to participate in research?

## SUGGESTED FURTHER READING

### Books

Armstrong, M. *Practical Nursing Management*. Edward Arnold, London, 1981.

Goldstone, L. A. *Statistics in the Management of Nursing Services*. Churchill Livingstone, London, 1981.

Hockey, L. (Ed.). *Current Issues in Nursing*. Recent Advances in Nursing Series, Churchill Livingstone, London, 1981.

Kron, T. *Management of Patient Care: Putting Leadership Skills to Work*. Holt-Saunders, New York, 1986.

Macleod Clark, J. and Hockey, L. *Research for Nursing: A Guide for the Enquiring Nurse*. HM&M, London, 1979.

Marriner, A. *Nursing Process: A Scientific Approach to Nursing Care*, 2nd edition. Mosby, New York, 1979.

Pyne, R. N. *Professional Discipline in Nursing*. Blackwell Scientific, Oxford, 1981.

Royal College of Nursing. *Ethics Related to Research in Nursing*. RCN. London, 1977.

United Kingdom Central Council for Nursing, Midwifery and Health Visiting, *Code of Professional Conduct*, 2nd edition. UKCC, London, 1984.

### Bibliographies and Abstracts

Cumulative Index to Nursing and Allied Health Literature
Hospital Abstracts
Index Medicus
International Nursing Index
Nursing Research Abstracts

### Journals

*American Journal of Nursing*
*British Medical Journal*
*Health and Social Services Journal*
*Health Services Manpower Review*
*International Journal of Nursing Studies*
*Lancet*
*Journal of Advanced Nursing*
*Nurse Education Today*
*Nursing*
*Nursing Research*
*Nursing Times*

## POSTSCRIPT: RULE OF CONDUCT

Do all the good you can,
By all the means you can,
In all the ways you can,
In all the places you can,
At all the times you can,
To all the people you can,
As long as ever you can.

THURROCK TECHNICAL COLLEGE